NEVER
be a VICTIM

The Practice of Psychological Self-Defense

NEVER
be a VICTIM

Edward N. Ross, PhD

Hartley & Marks
PUBLISHERS

Published by

HARTLEY & MARKS PUBLISHERS INC.

P. O. Box 147   3661 West Broadway

Point Roberts, WA   Vancouver, BC

98281   V6R 2B8

Text © 1996 by Edward N. Ross

Illustrations © 1996 by HARTLEY & MARKS, INC.

Library of Congress Cataloging-in-Publication Data

Ross, Edward N., 1929–
     Never be a victim : the practice of psychological self-defense / Edward N. Ross
          p.   cm.
     Includes bibliographical references (p.   )
     ISBN 0-88179-115-6
          1. Crime prevention—United States. 2. Violent crimes—United States—
     Prevention. 3. Self-defense—United States.   I. Title.
     HV9950.R67   1996
     362.88—dc20   96-15765
                                                         CIP

Designed and typeset by The Typeworks
Set in MINION

Printed in the U.S.A.

Dedicated to my son, Bruce Evan, who inspired and encouraged me to write this book and provided many ideas that went into it, and for his continued input along the way.

Table of Contents

Introduction:
From Thomas J. Patire,
Self-Defense Expert

IT DOESN'T HAPPEN
THE WAY YOU THINK IT WILL

FOR MANY YEARS, I have watched and studied violent altercations on TV and in the movies, realizing that the public doesn't have a true view of the type of changes that happen to the human body during these events. Movies and books portray the attacks as heroic acts with the good guys coming out with the least injuries, never giving the violent act a second thought. This is a fallacy and the reality of violent altercations has never been brought to light.

I am going to give you a first-hand look at what goes on in your body and mind during the use of physical force while defending yourself. I will begin with a brief background of myself, so you may have a better insight into how violence has long played a role in my life.

I was born, raised and am still living in a small New Jersey borough—a community which has some very rough areas. I have had my share of street fights, and realized early in my youth that no one wins a fight. No matter what happens, both parties usually sustain some type of injury.

I joined a martial arts class at a young age, and experimented with different styles until I found the one that fit my personality. It was a complete form of martial arts, taught by a unique instructor. This gentleman gave me his personal insight into the real world of violence, and prepared me for what I call the mind and body conflict. Because, when faced with a life-and-death situation, the mind and body must not be in conflict. They must work together.

Working in many famous night clubs as a security person gave me the chance to use my physical skills when situations got out of hand. From there I intensified my training and moved on to bodyguard work in government, celebrity and corporate sectors. This type of work always deals with a high-stress environment and instant decisions, where violence sometimes becomes your only exit to safety. It involves thorough and constant training in many areas. A true bodyguard is not only a proficient fighter, he is an expert marksman, an evasive driver, and a very knowledgeable first-aider. He must also be aware of the various laws and types of liability in each of the states and countries he is traveling through.

What follows is an in-depth look at violence as seen through the eyes of a professional. I will take you through each individual step as it happens, and explain the thought process that is required to adapt, defend, and escape the assault.

The scenario: You are in a dangerous area. You get into a situation of a one-on-one assault, and you have no way out except to use physical force. The encounter begins. Here is how you feel physically, emotionally, and psychologically.

AN EXPERT'S EXPERIENCE OF VIOLENCE

The Lead-Up

Physical   As you see the altercation approaching your heart is racing, your adrenaline is pumping. Your vision becomes tunneled and your nerves taut. Your mind is fighting the reaction as you are wondering what to do first. You are sick to your stomach and your body begins to feel weak. Nerves begin to take over and twitching facial muscles act up. Your skin turns pale and your breathing gets deeper. Your limbs feel weak and your body feels like a dead weight.

Emotional   Your emotions are a mix of anger and fear. Your feelings are starting to get the best of you. You want to act out of impulsiveness but your mind knows better. You are trying to keep your emotions at bay. You know that if they go haywire your physical energy will be depleted. This would weaken your body before the struggle has even begun.

Psychological As the opponent approaches you, you clear your mind of all negative thoughts. They are replaced with positive thoughts of confidence and assertiveness. You instill the belief in your own superiority over the person who is trying to violate your right to life. It is either you or him. You pick the direct path to the quickest end that would be in your favor.

The Assault

Physical Reaction You are about to be struck. Your hands rise in automatic defense. The strike rattles your body even though it was blocked. You counter with a defensive strike, and your mind and senses turn into an emotional rage. You don't know whether to scream, cry, or start yelling. Your body counters again and again until the attacker is disabled. You look at the person lying on the ground. Your body is totally weakened, your legs are like rubber, your upper limbs are numb. As you move farther and farther away, a queasiness fills your stomach.

Emotional Reaction As your rights begin to be violated you feel an instant dislike or hatred for the attacker. He has created a fury within you that brings out the violent side that lurks in all of us. You want to take all your frustrations out on this victimizer, because he had the nerve to violate you with physical force.

Psychological Reaction Your mind has found the center line: the trained reaction of the body and mind to protect the body under these conditions. The thought process focuses on defense to whatever extreme point is needed to neutralize the situation.

The Immediate Aftermath

Physical Reaction You are now away from the scene and resting in your car. You glance at your watch and realize the altercation that you thought took minutes only took seconds. Your body is totally drained of physical strength. You check for injuries and start feeling the aches and pains as the numbness wears off your body. Your body returns to normal. Your vision is clear and your hearing is sound. Breathing and heartbeat resume their normal pattern. You check your physical state and find minor cuts and bruises, but you realize your overall condition is good.

Emotional Reaction   You don't know whether to laugh or cry. You feel an emptiness inside, caused by the question of whether you acted appropriately. You wonder if it is over, or if this person will enter your life again somewhere in the future. You think about all that could have happened if the circumstances had been different. If a weapon was involved, you wonder how you avoided it. You have wandering thoughts about the attacker's background and what this person could be about. When things finally settle down you realize that everything worked in the proper sequence for keeping yourself safe and protected.

Psychological Reaction   Your mind made a decision to act in a scenario that you were trained for. Your confidence combined with your thought process reacted to an extremely high-pressure situation. The mind made the right decisions and the body answered accordingly. You come to the decision that you had no other choice. You are at peace with yourself. It was either you or him.

ANGER AND SURVIVAL

There are many emotions, reactions, feelings, and physical attributes people must realize are involved when they undergo and survive a life-and-death ordeal. It is true that different personality types will influence the responses to the situation at hand, but in a life-and-death situation, the only choice is survival. Even though personalities may vary tremendously, behavior can be altered in a time of need.

Through my travels as a professional bodyguard, and also as a martial arts instructor to many Fortune 500 companies, I have had the privilege of interviewing many types of victims. These victims came from different types of backgrounds, and were of different races, ages, genders, and sizes. Their outlooks on life varied according to their geographical location, their philosophies, and their social environments. All agreed that when there was no other alternative during their ordeal, they focused on using some type of aggression to help make their exit to safety. They yelled or screamed to attract attention, disabled their attacker by clawing, biting, kicking, or pounding, and ran to safety when they saw a clear escape.

SOME COMMON RISK FACTORS

I have come to the conclusion that even though people are targeted at random, there are some common factors that contribute to their victimization. One is location. There is the geographical area, the individual's destination, the place of origin, and the number of isolation zones. It is a known fact that certain types of areas are more likely to encompass certain criminal elements. For example, a shopping center gives a robber a variety of victims, due to the large number of people that frequent the area. The types of stores can differentiate the average-income person from the above-average, just by the store they shop in. Location also involves the road the person travels on, and the area chosen for parking. It can help car-jackers make sure their victim can't escape them when they try to steal a vehicle. The place of origin refers to the initial location of the assault, and how and why the victim was first spotted.

In isolation zones a person is not in clear view of other people, which provides the opportunity to isolate a victim for a one-on-one assault. Examples of this are alleyways, low-lit parking areas, and areas that you are not familiar with.

I have found that people are selected due to the first impression they make. Believe it or not, your demeanor and how you carry yourself can affect you as a potential victim. Body size and shape, gender, and all-round appearance are definite factors influencing any type of criminal activity. Very seldom do you hear of a person of significant size being manhandled, abused, raped, or mugged. Many rape victims were chosen due to their appearance, type of clothing, and body shape. This doesn't necessarily mean that rapists choose as their targets the best-shaped figures. In essence, they choose according to their own personal preference.

Many targeted victims were robbed or mugged because of the way they exposed their money while shopping or the way they overexposed the jewelry on their persons. Flashy jewelry, whether real or costume, can be a lucrative target to someone in need of cash. The best way to become less of a target is to dress "down." Rings should be turned to the inside of the palm so only the band is exposed, not the gems. Bracelets should be worn to the inside of the wrist, while necklaces should be worn out of sight, inside the dress or shirt. I agree that jewelry is a thing of beauty and does deserve to be shown off. However, keeping it hidden until you arrive at your destination can lower the odds of your becoming a victim.

The most important way to reduce your risk of becoming the chosen target is to carry yourself with the utmost confidence. Walk directly to your destination, keeping your head up and your eyes scanning the general area. Be attentive and alert, and never underestimate any potential situation. A recent survey of state convicts reported that they said they targeted people they knew would not struggle, or people they thought would not chase them after they had stolen their purse or wallet. When asked how they picked their targets one man said, "I watched how they walked. If they seemed like they had no energy and they looked out of shape, they were mine." All agreed that they were less likely to challenge someone projecting an aura of confidence and self-preservation. Expect the unexpected, and never give anyone the benefit of the doubt.

Conclusion

What I have said about the way the body reacts under duress, and what is experienced in the mind while being attacked, is based on my interviews of many people who had little or no self-defense training. What happened to them was terrifying but real, and will haunt them every day of their lives. Some of us choose to ignore random violence, and some of us are paranoid about it, but I believe it is part of life. Expect it and be ready for it, but don't let thoughts of becoming victimized control you.

Thomas J. Patire

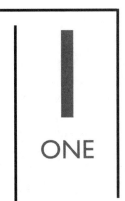

The Truth About Violence

ONE

W E ARE LIVING in a world where violence is taken for granted. For years we have known that the United States is becoming an increasingly violent place in which to live. Themes of violence have long been prevalent in television and motion pictures, and violence in the home is commonplace at all socioeconomic levels.

The United States has been identified as a culture of violence, within which a subculture exists that contributes to the high rates of violence compared to other developed nations. Many analysts have observed that violence is built into every aspect of American society, beginning with the use of physical force as the resource to rely on when we are children if all other approaches seem to fail.

The victimization of human beings by human beings is now so out of control that fear has gripped the young, middle-aged, and elderly on an equal basis. It is not uncommon to hear strong, burly men express fear for their well-being when approaching a few youths who appear to be looking for trouble. Years ago, an adult would have said without hesitation, "Be on your way, sonny" or "Go home to your mother." Now one thinks twice before daring to say anything, frightened that it may cause a knife, gun, or other weapon to be brandished.

OUR SURVIVAL ATTITUDES

Few of us think of ourselves as potential victims of an attack before anything has happened to us. Rather, we feel that we are less apt than most people to become victims of a crime. This belief has been labeled "unique invulnerability." If we are attacked, we discover we must cope both with the direct consequences of the experience, and with the loss of our feeling of invulnerability. We also feel more at risk about our future vulnerability, and all these fears add to our existing feelings of stress following the initial victimization.

When addressing woman's groups I always ask the question, "If you were in the process of a rape attack and had an open opportunity to gouge your assailant's eyes, could you do it?" A conservative estimate is that at least 95 percent of the women respond either with an outright "No," or will say such things as, "I doubt it," "I don't think so," "It would go against my nature," and so on. Even if I add the question, "If you were pretty certain you might be killed?" the percentage of responses remain unchanged. There is not much variation in type and percentage of responses if I substitute squeezing the testicles for gouging the eyes. Now if a woman feels this way in the safety of a lecture hall, it is likely that she would not be able to do any of these things if attacked.

To some people the ability to be verbally and physically assertive comes naturally. For others—women more so than men—it is not easy. But this is something that can be learned. Many patients ask me, "What should I say/do when John says/does such and such?" When I discuss their options with them, they usually respond with something like, "Gee, that sounds so easy, why didn't I think of it?" or, "How will I ever remember these things?" When I tell them that they will be able to learn how to think on their feet without becoming flustered, rattled, and blocked, I assure them that they will have to take my word for now, until they see for themselves. Before long, they are saying such things to me as, "I'm getting there, it's getting easier, and I'm learning." As you develop the "survival attitude" (discussed in Chapter 2), you will notice many things happening. Behavioral and psychological changes will begin taking place in your relationships with your spouse, work associates, friends—for that matter everyone with whom you associate.

WHOM THIS BOOK IS FOR

If you believe that you can do more than you are already doing to be better prepared, this book is for you. If you believe there must be a better way to protect yourself, this book is for you. If you believe that you should take more responsibility for your own survival because you cannot totally depend upon law enforcement, community programs, or the conventional methods in use, this book is for you.

As you learn how defensive survival psychology is combined with a specific method of response, these beliefs will be strengthened. I can assure you of this for two reasons. First, because defensive survival psychology is based upon well-established psychological theory and behavioral observations. Second, because it has been clearly shown that when the principles of defensive survival psychology are used together with certain techniques anxiety is overcome, attitudes improve, and positive changes in behavior are brought about. (See Recommended Reading.)

THROUGH THE BACK DOOR

Though I am a psychologist specializing in prevention, treatment, and education in the areas of violence, abuse, victimization, and crime prevention, I did not set out to make this my specialty. It found me.

For the past thirty years of practice, I have worked with a number of people in abusive relationships requiring treatment—as have many practitioners. However, several years ago, more of them began finding their way to me—victims of domestic violence, sexual abuse, crime, and other varieties of violence.

In working with them, I came to see that our methods, approaches, and techniques were woefully in need of updating. Moreover, preventive approaches have been almost nonexistent. What has been ignored is the fact that violence is both physical and psychological in nature. All acts of violence are motivated by psychological factors, and all acts of violence produce both physical and psychological consequences. This is why prevention, treatment, and survival must be dealt with on both these levels.

Two very vivid examples always stand out in my mind. I had been working with a middle-aged woman with anxiety and intermittent periods of depression for about a year and a half, when one day out of the blue she told me that she had been raped when in her early twenties. I asked her if she had ever reported it to the police, or had gone to any

Our lives are so saturated with crime reports and statistics that we are conditioned to accept violence as an everyday part of our society.

support groups, or contacted a rape crisis center. To all of these questions she answered "No."

She said that after the wealth of information she had been exposed to from reading, the radio, and television, she did not care for the way rape victims were treated by the police, or the courts, or looked upon by society, and felt she knew as much as anyone could tell her about the trauma she had experienced and what she could expect. She then described her symptoms, comparing them to what is known as "rape trauma syndrome." She related the way she had coped with the trauma, and her rehabilitative process. And she ended by stating that because all rape victims are treated in the same general manner, she had never done anything about it.

She had managed to cope with the rape by ignoring it, by not giving any credence to its existence. This psychological mechanism, known as denial, is often used by rape victims, among others. But what she was saying was true. She was describing what has been called "secondary victimization"—the ways law enforcement, the judicial system, and society contribute to making the rape victim feel ashamed, blamed, and stigmatized.

The second example concerns a man in his mid-forties who was referred to me by his family physician after being assaulted. Getting out of his car, he was approached by two youths, one of whom grabbed him from behind, while the other proceeded to go through his pockets. After they got what they wanted, he was knocked down and they fled. Fortunately he was not seriously hurt.

But a few weeks later, he began having a variety of unrelated physical symptoms: frequent headaches, stomach cramps, and periods of impotence. He was becoming easily irritated, even though he was generally a very calm and tolerant person. He returned to his doctor, and after a thorough examination was found to be free of any physiological reasons for his symptoms. The physician felt they were due to psychological or emotional causes.

I began seeing this man on a regular basis, and it became evident that he was feeling a tremendous amount of anger which he could not express. As treatment progressed, the reasons surfaced. He had grown up in a family with an abusive father who often hit his mother. Hating the repeated violent anger as well as the physical aggression that accompanied it, he vowed never to be like his father. Instead, he became a nonassertive, docile, conforming adult, unable to show any anger. So much so, that the appropriate anger or assertiveness necessary to discipline his own children became a distasteful and sometimes impossible chore. Now he was faced with an inordinate amount of anger and a desire for revenge and retribution. He could not vent these feelings. Instead they were pent up and produced the physical (psychosomatic) symptoms.

Concurrent with psychotherapy, he enrolled in a program to learn self-defense skills, and was ultimately able to resolve his repressed anger, and his inability to express his feelings appropriately.

A BETTER WAY

Every act of our lives is the sum of many determinants. Every act of behavior, every response, is unique to the individual who produces it. These individual differences have special meaning for each victim of violence and must be understood in terms of the anxieties they experience.

To persist in using methods of treatment and prevention without knowing if they are suitable for everyone is like putting a group of children with a wide range of IQs, chronological ages, and diverse cultural backgrounds into the same class, and expecting them to all learn adequately and at the same rate with the same teaching techniques.

That there are feelings of guilt and vulnerability accompanied by a lack of confidence in those who have been attacked is to be expected. No matter how unprovoked, most victims of violence feel a certain amount of guilt about what has happened to them. They second-guess themselves about things they may have done wrong, or could have done differently, and they experience other elements of self-blame. They feel more vulnerable after a trauma and their self-confidence is considerably shaken.

But a very serious pattern that previously had gone unnoticed by me began occurring all too often to be considered mere chance. After many of these disturbing feelings were thought to have been resolved during the rehabilitative treatment, they again surfaced, now completely unrelated to the assault, or to any other known previous trauma. They emerged as feelings which had been either repressed (painful past experiences kept hidden from one's awareness) or suppressed (deliberately forgotten), and now appeared as part of the survivor's personality.

When I checked my observations with numerous colleagues in research, teaching, and private practice, all were in agreement. Their experiences were similar, and no one, including myself, had put all these elements together.

For the majority of people, abuse and victimization result in physical as well as psychological trauma. Standard approaches have not been as effective as possible because the insult to the body has been ignored. For this reason prevention and treatment needs are unique, and the techniques, methods, and goals must take into account both mind (the psychological) and body (the physical).

This is shown dramatically in the following true story.

In 1984 Kathy Holub, a California journalist, was raped in her own house. She later wrote a chronicle of the circumstances and aftermath of this horrible event for her paper. She wrote that after the rape, she had rejected everyone's suggestions that she take a self-defense course. But several years later, when she went to New York, just eight months after the highly publicized rape of a Central Park jogger, she spent the entire visit in terror listening to all her friends talk about crime. Years before, she had read about a self-defense training program designed especially for women (Model Mugging). She had rejected this out of hand, since, as she wrote, attacking a man even in self-defense contradicted everything she had been taught about being female. She believed that putting the knee to the groin was an unnatural act and quite unthinkable. These feelings were not surprising, in fact they were quite natural, since women are taught to believe that men are their protectors, and that physical aggression and fighting are unfeminine. Well, more than five years later she did enroll in Model Mugging, and an interesting thing happened. In Holub's words:

> In retrospect, I believe that the rape was somehow "stored"
> in my body until I was ready to face it emotionally. It was almost as if the memory of the attack flowed directly into my

joints and got stuck there. That's the best way I can explain the denial I managed to sustain for the next five years. I walked around like a frozen person: functional, fortunately—able to go to work every day—but largely insulated from my emotions and totally disconnected from my body, which I cloaked in the baggiest garments I could find. Although I really did expect the rape to come up as a topic in therapy, it never did. This was the most baffling of all. When it came to the rape, I drew a blank.

The release valve came from an unlikely quarter, and it was sudden. One day in Model Mugging I popped my heel hard into my instructor's groin. THWOCK! It was a perfect hit. I heard the cracking sound of my foot against the heavy padding, I felt the impact, I saw my heel slam into its target, and suddenly I was so angry I wanted to kill the man. That was the beginning of my thawing-out process. And I must say it was a frightening process at first. My emotions appalled me; I did not want to feel them. Fortunately, Model Mugging is designed to help with precisely this difficulty, and every time I confronted strong emotions during the training, my instructors encouraged me to see it as a breakthrough. Gradually I got used to these feelings and even accepted them as normal. That, in turn, helped me integrate the fact of rape into my life.

Holub added that now she understood why simply talking about the assault had never worked.

As a result of all this I started to concentrate more on the preventive and survival aspects of victimizing and life-threatening experiences by working with the mind/body connection, and began developing a new way of looking at this whole area. Mental health professionals have been receptive to this new approach, and anyone can easily understand how it can be incorporated into the protective aspects of everyday living.

I call this new area of psychology defensive survival psychology.

2
TWO

Defensive Survival Psychology: The Mind/Body Connection

WHEN I BEGAN researching the relationship between the mind and the body in relation to treating and preventing abuse and victimization, the medical profession was just beginning to look into the possibility that one's physical health, and even more important, one's entire immune system, might be affected by this interaction.

Since then, a new area of medicine has been identified and given the name psychoneuroimmunology (PNI). It is exploding with new scientific data proving that certain kinds of mental activity actually do cause an increase in disease-fighting cells within the body. For instance, patients with serious illnesses, even terminal diseases, have experienced a reversal or remission of the disease when they have adopted positive mental attitudes, and engaged in certain prescribed mental activities along with their medical treatments. This has been attributed to the body's ability to strengthen its immune system, its disease-fighting cells. A modern revival is taking place of the age-old beliefs that a strong connection exists between psychology and physiology. This is not surprising when psychology has been called the oldest form of medicine.

THE POWER OF OUR MIND

Although the mind/body connection has a long and venerable history, it is only recently that western modern medicine has been attempting to try and catch up with what eastern cultures and some indigenous populations have been aware of for centuries—that there seem to be no limits to the power of our mind.

This is why Socrates said that there is no illness of the body apart from the mind, and why Dr. Albert Schweitzer described the reasons for the witch doctor's success, explaining that it is no different from the success of all doctors. By carrying his own witch doctor within himself, the patient has the power that enables him to do his work.

In the field of mental health, Sigmund Freud long ago demonstrated how emotional conditions can produce dramatic physiological changes, such as blindness and paralysis. Problems deeply buried in the unconscious were observed to produce physical symptoms which could be removed by hypnosis.

Recognizing this link between mind and body, an increasing number of modern-day physicians have begun to study the relationship between the mind and the immune system, and have started to treat disease by treating the mind and body as a single unit, rather than two separate entities. Dr. O. Carl Simonton, a radiologist specializing in cancer treatment and author of *Getting Well Again*, has successfully been using imagery with his patients since 1965. Dr. Bernie Siegel, author of *Love, Medicine, and Miracles*, is a cancer surgeon who utilizes guided imagery in the treatment of cancer. Dr. Dean Ornish, author of *Dr. Dean Ornish's Program for Reversing Heart Disease*, is a cardiologist who uses visualization with cardiac patients, and Dr. Martin Rossman, who wrote *Healing Yourself*, uses imagery in his general practice. Dr. Andrew Weil, author of *Natural Health, Natural Medicine*, is another of the many who are combining medical with psychological treatments.

Many techniques used in the treatment of illness are based on the mind/body interaction.

With hypnosis the mind gains control over the body. This technique has been refined through the decades and is now used so frequently, and in such a variety of situations, that it is accepted by most people in a very matter-of-fact way.

Biofeedback produces bodily changes by training the mind to regulate physiological functions. It works like this. One is connected to a sensory apparatus which measures such bodily functions as skin temperature, blood pressure, and muscle contraction. This apparatus is also

Physicians are increasingly harnessing the power of the patient's mind to combat illness.

Our belief in the efficiency of drugs is a potent medicine in itself.

linked to a video screen which converts these functions to auditory signals and/or visual displays. One's measure of success in changing one's bodily functions is indicated by these signals.

Meditation has been proven to reduce the body's metabolic rate, thereby lowering blood pressure, the pulse rate, and the blood's stress hormone levels. It also raises the body's threshold for sensitivity to pain.

Psychosomatic illness is induced by the mind as a result of trauma or stress. There is no known organic cause for psychosomatic symptoms, but they nevertheless are produced by physiological changes accompanying emotional states. Even when there is a physical cause for a person's illness, such emotional states as fear and worry can aggravate the discomfort that goes with the illness.

And there is probably nothing that more clearly demonstrates the mind/body interaction than the effects of placebos on bodily function. Patients who receive nonmedical substances, like sugar pills, can show the disappearance of the symptoms of their disease, and a drastic reduction in pain. This is well-known as "the placebo effect."

FIGHT-OR-FLIGHT RESPONSE

This same mechanism occurs in the fight-or-flight response where the mind and body respond to an immediate threat of stress and danger. It is called the fight-or-flight response because the body prepares itself in the same protective ways for survival to all perceived danger. This danger can be physical or emotional, and the preparation can be to fight or run. Threats can range from a fear of being physically hurt to a fear of being emotionally rejected.

The following physiological reactions to stress help to explain the fight-or-flight response. They prepare the body to physically survive a life-threatening event. But do not forget, it is your state of mind at the time which is telling your body what to do, and it is also your state of mind which will determine your behavior. Dr. Ornish describes the fight-or-flight response as involving the following changes.

✔*Our muscles begin to contract, thereby fortifying our "body armor." We are more protected from bodily injury.*

✔ *Our metabolism speeds up, providing more strength and energy with which to fight or run. Both our heart rate and the amount of blood pumped with each beat increase.*

✔ *Our rate of breathing begins to increase, providing more oxygen to do battle or to run from danger.*

✔ *Our digestive system begins to shut down, diverting more blood and energy to the large muscles needed to fight or run.*

✔ *The pupils of our eyes begin to dilate, aiding vision. Other senses such as hearing also become heightened.*

✔ *We feel an urge to urinate and move the bowels, to reduce the danger of infection if abdominal injury should occur.*

✔ *Arteries in our arms and legs begin to constrict, so that less blood will be lost if we become wounded or injured. (You may notice that your hands get cold during times of stress, which is the principle behind the "stress cards" in which the color of the card you hold begins to change as you become more relaxed.)*

✔ *Our blood clots more quickly, so we'll lose less blood if we become wounded or injured.*

OUR MIND/BODY INTERACTION AND ACHIEVEMENTS

It should not be surprising then to conclude that something that can produce drastic physiological changes can also work to help us accomplish many other things.

There is no doubt that this is true. There are numerous verified stories of people who have accomplished physical and psychological acts of heroism and courage in the face of danger, and performed superhuman feats of endurance which under normal conditions would have been impossible. These range from women who have lifted cars and pulled trapped children from beneath them, to an eighty-two-year-old Chinese Ch'i Kung master who with his bare forehead drove an eight-inch nail through a board four inches thick.

When faced with a life-and-death situation, the mind and body must work together.

We can learn to use our minds to overcome fear, pain and suffering.

☒ ORIGINAL
☐ SUPPLEMENT

GENERAL INCIDENT REPORT
SOUTHGATE POLICE DEPARTMENT

PAGE 1 OF 4 X

INCIDENT NO.	REPORTING OFFICER	SERIAL 1	SERIAL 2	REPORT TIME & DATE	OCCURRED BETWEEN TIME-DATE	OCCURRED ON TIME-DATE
80-013086	PIQUARD	045		1800 10-29-80	1500—1530	10/29/8

INCIDENT TYPE	CLASSIFICATION	INCIDENT ADDRESS		DISTRICT
CITIZEN RESCUE	9010	HELEN + WESLEY (N.W. CORNER)		A 32

REPORT TAKEN AT ☒ SCENE ☐ STAT ☐ PHONE ☐ OTHER

	NAME	R/S	D.O.B.	INVOLVEMENT	ARRESTED	HOME PHONE	BUS. PHONE
A	LEMERAND, ARNOND	W/M	12-8-28	REP.	☐ Y ☒ N	281-0617	

ADDRESS: 12316 HELEN
EMPLOYER: PENNWALT
WORK HOURS:

	NAME	R/S	D.O.B.	INVOLVEMENT	ARRESTED	HOME PHONE	BUS. PHONE
B	VENDITTI, GUY	W/M	40		☐ Y ☒ N		371-638

ADDRESS: 41847 MAROLD, ST. HGTS.
EMPLOYER: PACENTRO CONST.
WORK HOURS:

	NAME	R/S	D.O.B.	INVOLVEMENT	ARRESTED	HOME PHONE	BUS. PHONE
C	TOTH, PHILIP ANDREW	W/M	3-27-75		☐ Y ☒ N	284-2091	

ADDRESS: 12690 AGNES
EMPLOYMENT: SHELTERS
WORK HOURS:

NARRATIVE USING WHO, WHAT, WHERE, WHEN, WHY.

    I WAS DISPATCHED TO HELEN + WESLEY REGARDING CONSTRUCTION MATERIALS POSING A HAZARD. UPON ARRIVAL I TALKED TO "A" WHO RELATED THE FOLLOWING:

    "A" CAME HOME FROM THE STORE AND FOUND "C" LYING ON GROUND WITH A SECTION OF SEWER PIPE LYING ACROSS HIS HEAD + NECK AREA. THERE WERE 2 HYSTERICAL YOUNG GIRLS THERE TRYING TO HELP THE BOY (GIRLS UNIDENTIFIED - LEFT AREA AFTERWARDS)

    APPARENTLY "C" HAD BEEN PLAYING (WITH OTHER KIDS) ON SEWER PIPES + OTHER CONST. MATERIALS ON THAT CORNER - THE SECTION OF SEWER PIPE IN QUESTION WAS PROPPED ON 4"x4" PIECES OF LUMBER BY ITSELF AND COULD BE ROLLED ALONG THE 4x4" BEAMS IF PUSHED HARD ENOUGH. IT WAS EVIDENT THAT THE BOY, "C", HAD FALLEN DOWN AND THE SEWER PIPE SECTION ROLLED DOWN TO THE STUDS AT

FOLLOW-UP ASSIGNED TO	SERIAL	SQUAD	ASSIGN. DATE	VALUE ☐ S ☐ R	CURRENCY	JEWELRY	CLOTHING
	064	11			A	B	C

DISPOSITION DATE	DISPOSITION	RECLASSIFICATION	LOC. STL. M.V.	OFFICE EQUIP.	T.V., RADIO, ETC.	FIREARMS
10/30/80	08		D	E	F	G

IF '02' DISPOSITION

	ADULTS	JUVENILES	HOUSEHOLD	CONSUMABLE	LIVESTOCK	MISC.
			H		J	K

LICENSE	STATE	NUMBER	V.I.N.	LEIN ☐ E ☐ R	TIME	DATE	BY WHOM

CAR	MAKE	MODEL	STYLE	COLOR	OFFICER'S SIGNATURE	REVIEWED BY

INCIDENT NUMBER: 80-013086

.6 SPD 6/80

D.3. – ASSIGNMENT

⊠ ORIGINAL
☐ SUPPLEMENT

GENERAL INCIDENT REPORT
SOUTHGATE POLICE DEPARTMENT

PAGE _2_ OF _4_ X ☐ Y
DB ⊠ N

INCIDENT NO. 80-013086

INCIDENT TYPE RESCUE   CLASSIFICATION 9010

NARRATIVE USING WHO, WHAT, WHERE, WHEN, WHY.

ENDS of 4"x4"'s passing over "C"'s body and coming to rest on "C" head and neck trapping him to the ground. "A" states that upon his arrival "C" was semi concious and blue in the face. Seeing that time was crucial "A" simply lifted one end of the pipe section and told the girls to drag the boy, "C", out to safety "A" found out from "C" where he lived (on Agnes) and carried "C" home + T.O.T. mom.

✱ Note - I tried to lift the same pipe section + was unable to budge same - I was informed by "B", a const. employee, that these pipe sections, of about 15-20 ft. in length, weigh around 1800 lbs. apiece. "A" also tried to lift it again and was unable to a second time.

I explained what happened to "B" and he secured the pipe length the best he could making it harder

NARRATIVE USING WHO, WHAT, WHERE, WHEN, WHY.

to move it. (put stop blocks on both sides of pipe) "B" wasn't surprised that the boy was trapped - says kids are constantly trying to roll the pipes and he has had to come out at night sev. times, to put them back on the easement after kids rolled them in the street.

I talked to "C" mother and Dr. David Kreske, Allen Park (ph # 386-1100) who admitted "C" into O.A. Hosp. for observation. "C" has a concussion, abrasions and some slight hemorraging of surface capillaries on face but appears to be O.K. - both mother and doctor acknowledge that "A" undoubtealy saved "C" life by his quick actions and sudden super-human strength.

We experience a multitude of thoughts, emotions and physical changes during a life-and-death ordeal.

From an official police report of a case of extraordinary strength mobilized in a severe crisis situation.

We must think positive thoughts in order to effect positive changes.

In 1980 the Boston Globe ran a story about a fifty-six-year-old man who, because of a heart attack suffered six years earlier, was averse to lifting heavy objects. But that week, when a five-year-old youngster was trapped under a cast-iron pipe near a playground, he easily lifted the pipe and saved the child's life. He estimated the weight of the pipe to be around three or four hundred pounds. The actual weight was nearly a ton (two thousand pounds). Afterwards, this man, his grown sons, reporters, and police all tried to lift the pipe but were unable to do so.

There are many examples of those who have been able to "psyche out" or influence others by manipulating their own physiological processes, their thoughts and emotions. There are those who have had the power to "cast a spell" over an opponent, or audience, and stories of athletes, martial artists, samurai warriors, and others who at certain times have been totally immune to pain while possessed of extraordinary strength, energy, power, speed, balance, acute sensory perception, and extrasensory abilities. These skills enabled them to perform unbelievably difficult acts with ease, and to achieve such a state of invulnerability that they could not be harmed.

We know also of ritual fire walks on hot coals which take place in some lands. There is the yogi who sits on a bed of nails and feels no pain, or who allows himself to be buried alive for days to test the limits of self-mastery and the fakir who thrusts metal spikes through his tongue, neck, and stomach with no accompanying bleeding or pain.

Tibetan priests have been observed to sit naked in the snow and to dry out ice-cold water-soaked sheets that were wrapped around them with just the power of the heat generated from their bodies. These adepts could sit for hours at a time, actually melting the snow encircling them. They created bodily heat by visualizing a sun in certain nerve junctions of their bodies, thereby producing "psychic" heat.

In the 1930s, studies took place in the Soviet Union concerning the effects of visualization on the control of bodily functions. A research psychologist (Dr. A. R. Luria) demonstrated that a subject was able to increase his heart rate by imagining himself running after a train that had just pulled out, and to decrease his heart rate by imagining himself lying in bed perfectly still trying to fall asleep. He could raise the temperature in one hand by imagining that hand on a hot stove, and decrease the temperature in his other hand by imagining that he was squeezing a piece of ice. He could also alter the time it took for the pupils of his eyes to adapt to the dark by visualizing light variations.

Dramatic? Indeed it is—but all very real.

HOW BELIEF CAN CAUSE PHYSICAL CHANGES

To better understand this bodily drama in action, we can study the placebo effect. Placebos have been used since the time of Hippocrates. They are drugs only in the loosest sense of the word, because they can be merely sugar pills, or for that matter, capsules filled with parsley, garlic, oregano, or whatever. Such a pill or capsule is given the role of a remedy, or a medication when it is prescribed by a physician. When it does what the drug it mimics was designed to do, it is called a placebo.

There are many well-documented stories of patients who have almost miraculously rallied from a terminal illness after taking "medications" which were, in actuality, placebos. Dr. Siegel cites a case of a terminally ill cancer patient who had heard of a new drug called Krebiozen which was being evaluated at the clinic he was in. It was being administered only to patients who were expected to live at least three to six months, and this patient didn't qualify. Still, after begging and pleading, he received an initial injection. His physical condition improved almost immediately, the size of his tumors were reduced to half their size in a few days, and he had renewed vigor. This single injection was followed by more, and within ten days practically all signs of the disease had disappeared. Within two months, there were news reports questioning the benefits of this drug. When this reached his ears, he began to lose faith, and two months of practically perfect health gave way to the relapsed original state. But his doctor decided to tell the patient that the original drug shipment was defective, and now a new and potent batch was on its way. A few days were permitted to pass and the patient's anticipation of recovery had now become exceedingly strong. After receiving the new injection (of fresh water) the results were more startling than the first time, and the patient became symptom-free for over two months. But then the American Medical

Optimistic people generally enjoy stronger bodies and healthier lives.

In order to walk tall and strong you must think tall and strong.

Association announced that Krebiozen had absolutely no worth as a cancer-treating drug, and the patient, now out of the hospital, was re-admitted and died within two days.

In experiments where patients were given placebos and told what this "medication" was supposed to do, together with possible side effects, these predicted effects were duplicated. Studies have shown placebos to be 77 percent as effective as morphine in the relief of postoperative pain, and that as the pain becomes more severe, the placebo increases in effectiveness. With arthritics, placebos have been shown to be as beneficial as the conventional anti-arthritic drugs such as aspirin and cortisone. They have, in addition, accounted for improvements in eating, sleeping, and elimination in these patients. Heroin addicts who have received injectable placebos exhibited the same response as if they were taking the real drug, including withdrawal effects when the placebo was stopped.

Treating warts with a brightly colored inert dye, which patients believed contained a powerful medication, proved to be as effective as surgical removal. This was thought to be due to changes in the skin's physiology in response to the emotional effects of the placebo, which made it impossible for the warts to continue to thrive.

In people with a variety of ailments ranging from nausea to the common cold, up to 40 percent have reported a lessening of symptoms or a complete cure after taking placebos.

So why does a placebo do what it does when it really "does" nothing, in the sense that you and I understand the meaning of the verb "to do"? It is because of belief. For this same reason medicine men were effective and voodoo curses worked because witch doctors were believed to have the powers that made them work.

A psychologist who studies voodoo deaths among Caribbean people concluded that it is the victim's faith which causes death. His explanation for the phenomenon is that the victim, convinced of the hex and its power, becomes helpless. It is a kind of learned helplessness which takes over, compliantly leading the victim to a resigned death.

Dr. Jerome Frank, a well-known psychiatrist, has drawn an analogy between the positive actions of a placebo and the negative mechanism of taboo death. The placebo, a symbol of healing, triggers a healing visualization in the patient, the effectiveness of the visualization being strengthened by the authority of the doctor administering the drug. In the case of death caused by a curse or spell, he hypothesizes that there is a prolonged over-stimulation of the adrenal glands resulting from a fear-induced over-activity of the vagus nerve which stimulates the heart.

All this means that every one of us has untapped resources and skills that can be developed. It points to our ability to use our mind/body relation the way it was meant to be used, both in everyday living, and to help us prevent—and even survive—a life-threatening situation. It becomes our own psychological edge—but only if we believe.

This togetherness of mind and body is the underlying premise and basic cornerstone of defensive survival psychology, and depends upon mind/body harmony.

A MIND/BODY IMBALANCE AFFECTS OUR ACHIEVEMENT

In order for us to feel good about ourselves we must feel good all over. But when our mind and body are in a state of imbalance, we feel a sense of unease, discomfort, and dissatisfaction. We cannot feel emotionally confident and assured if we feel physically afraid and vulnerable, and we cannot feel physically competent and adequate if we feel emotionally insecure and incapable, and are having serious self-doubts.

If we minimize the extent to which this mind/body harmony influences the way we will behave under life-threatening circumstances, we do ourselves a grave injustice. I like to think of the mind/body connection as mind/body synergism. When mind and body are in tune, in harmony and in balance, they enhance one another, enabling each to function at optimal levels. There is a principle called homeostasis which explains that a stable and consistent balance must be maintained within our body if we are to function adequately from day to day. When certain stressful events occur which disrupt this balance, negative and uncomfortable experiences occur, which in turn motivate us to try to cope, and re-establish this balance. When we are unable to effectively use previously learned coping behaviors, as in rape or other life-threatening and traumatic situations, an emotional crisis may result.

When we feel confident both physically and psychologically, this is

All the physical strength and expert manoeuvres in the world are useless if the mind is not prepared.

Taking responsibility for your feelings and your abilities is the first step in self-defense.

unmistakably communicated to others, just as when we feel weak or afraid. This is conveyed through our way of speaking, our attire, general attitude, our energy levels, awareness, and in many other ways. These feelings are integrally related to our susceptibility to assault, and our ability to survive a life-or-death situation.

The only way we can survive violence is to prepare ourselves physically and psychologically, and be aware of our surroundings. This does not simply involve being able to physically repel an attacker. It involves being psychologically ready and able to do anything and everything in order to survive.

Some black-belt martial artists who have demonstrated expert mechanical defense skills in the gymnasium or in tournament competition have frozen in panic when faced with a life-threatening situation on the street. This is why learning defensive skills alone is not the answer. Instead, what is needed is emotional readiness, the state of freedom from those personality problems which might block our ability to respond successfully and do without compunction anything and everything necessary to survive.

Readying oneself to confront a situation is commonly referred to as "psyching oneself up." This has also been called our mind-set, or psychological set, or preparatory set. It is what causes physiological changes to occur, similar to the fight-or-flight response. I mention these here because they are used later on in the book.

Emotional readiness is dependent upon many feelings and attitudes, and you must be emotionally ready and able to use your body to respond. When confronted with the panic of a traumatic life-threatening situation, your body may be prepared for action, but your mind may not. Faced with this kind of paralyzing fear, it is important not to let a "mental stall" occur which would sabotage the body's ability to respond. In this state of tension, people are also apt to act inappropriately. For example, an overly physically aggressive person might lash out against an attacker in an excitable frenzy, and in the process do the wrong thing.

Properly preparing yourself also involves recognizing and accepting the fact that you may fall victim. By assuming this cannot happen, we adopt a false sense of security and stop thinking in terms of our personal safety. This is the "it can't happen to me" syndrome.

Unless we can recognize the real dangers we may encounter and work to eliminate them, our odds for survival are greatly reduced. Holding on to the "it can't happen to me" belief can be deadly in a life-threatening situation, because this can prevent us from developing a survival attitude, the final cornerstone of defensive survival psychology.

LOCUS OF CONTROL

Another factor crucial to developing our "survival attitude" which is closely linked to the concept of self-reliance is called "locus of control." There are some of us who feel it is beyond our capacity to change the situations we find ourselves in, or certain events and circumstances that happen to us. Our feelings about ourselves, our abilities, and moods are viewed as dependent upon and originating from other persons or sources. Those of us who feel this way are more apt to place the responsibility for our predicament on these external factors, on someone or something other than ourselves, and are said to have a "high external locus of control."

Those of us who have a "high internal locus of control" feel that we are more responsible for circumstances that occur.

This concept is very important in the prevention and survival process because it looks at our behavior outside the context of blame. Blame can be counter-productive and destructive to all of us, and undermines the survival process.

Dr. Siegel has found that people who feel that they are in control (those with a high internal locus of control), have achieved remarkable medical recoveries from fatal, life-threatening illnesses. This is not to equate fighting one's disease (an attack from within) with fighting a bodily attack by an external assailant. However, it would seem that these kinds of people are more apt to be motivated towards developing a survival attitude.

Placing blame outside of yourself maintains a "victim" mentality.

The development of a "survival attitude" has been found to be necessary for creating an edge for yourself in any life-threatening situation. Do not lose sight of the fact that every attacker relies on specific things that give him his edge. He usually operates on his own turf, in familiar surroundings. He relies heavily on the elements of surprise, panic, and

Common sense is not something you are born with or without—it's a question of remaining focused.

fear in his victims, and frequently has a weapon. Below is a look at how we can go about providing our own edge.

HOW TO CREATE AN EDGE

There are five basic components to developing an edge.

1. Emotional Readiness and Preparatory Mindset. This state of mind is necessary for survival, and is one of the major cornerstones of effective self-defense.

2. Acute Sensory Awareness. This is what your senses convey in the process of assessing whether a danger is imagined, potential, or real. Sensory awareness deals with both social and environmental experiences. Social awareness involves sensitivity to individuals around us. It deals with who they are, why they are there, and how they are behaving. Environmental awareness involves sensitivity to your physical surroundings and how they might be used to your advantage or disadvantage.

3. High-Level Intuitive Skills. These are sometimes referred to as gut feelings, sixth sense, and ESP. In order for them to work on your behalf you must learn how to develop them and pay proper attention to them.

4. Formulating Your Strategies. Understanding the options at your disposal, and how to choose the most appropriate one. Only a limited number of tactics will be effective in each situation. They will be linked to the specific situation and environment, and your personal feelings about each one.

5. Protective Devices. These are simple, common objects which you might never think of as defensive weapons—things like pens, pencils, jewelry, books, kitchen utensils, belt buckles, etc. Women's purses and men's pockets contain many articles that could be used in self-defense.

Starting with the survival attitude, here is an explanation of what is involved in creating an edge.

The word "attitude" is defined as a set of beliefs and feelings towards some object or situation. Our attitudes are learned and can also be changed.

Consider the following statements.

✔*Law enforcement cannot adequately protect everyone.*

✔*Violence is increasing.*

✔*Everyone is becoming more at risk.*

✔*If you don't take some responsibility for your safety, no one else will.*

✔*The possibility exists that some day you could be targeted for an assault.*

How do you feel about these statements? Are they true? Well, of course they are. If you believe them, it should be easy for you to take the next step and start thinking in terms of surviving, so that the "survival attitude" becomes part of you.

Once you have done this, you have taken your first and most important step. You have made the commitment needed to make the preparations which will enable you to adopt your own style of survival. By style I mean what approach will work for you and make you feel comfortable and confident, rather than awkward and hesitant.

With your survival attitude in place, you can now turn to the requisites for developing your edge.

Emotional Readiness

This means being ready, willing, and able. Readiness can be learned, developed, and conditioned, so that when your inner call for help goes out, you will be able to respond as a total person. Your mind and body can be trained to think, feel, and act as one, automatically.

Establishing your "survival attitude" has put you in a different frame of mind, and motivated you to go forward.

To be emotionally ready means to be free of anxiety which can block you from thinking clearly and responding effectively—in some cases responding at all. One of the most successful ways of accomplishing this is through the use of relaxation techniques combined with guided imagery. (See Chapters 9 and 10.) As well as alleviating your anxiety, guided imagery allows you to stage your own "dress rehearsals," putting yourself in life-threatening situations and going through entire survival scenarios without leaving your living-room sofa.

Think of your senses as muscles: exercise them regularly and they'll become stronger.

Acute Sensory Awareness

Concentrating solely on your line of sight is a learned response—unlearn it by exercising your peripheral vision.

This area involves fine-tuning the senses and learning to use your sensory apparatus in unaccustomed ways.

Even if your visual, hearing, and olfactory apparatus is ultrasensitive, you must know how to make it work correctly for you. You cannot assume it is going to warn you of danger.

You have to make sure that you are looking for the important things. You must be certain that you are alert to your total surroundings, and then filter out what belongs there and what does not. In this way you will learn to see the forest and the trees.

In his book, Field Guide to Nature and Survival for Children, Tom Brown explains how to sharpen children's senses. He says that with practice, children are able to regain and sharpen the sensory awareness that has become dulled and atrophied, and to reverse damage caused by poorly used senses and acquired bad habits.

Most people, even those who are generally more observant than others, can be trained to further develop their visual discriminatory skills. The techniques Brown describes can be applied to adults as well as children.

Each of us knows the limitations of our visual and hearing capabilities. You know how good your near, far, and peripheral vision is, how well and how fast you accommodate to changing lighting conditions, and the methods that work best for you in compensating for your deficiencies.

This also holds true for hearing. You know how acute your hearing is, from what side (if any) you hear better, and what kinds of sounds pose the most or least difficulties.

To sharpen your individual senses you might want to try the following. It may also come in handy if one or more of your senses becomes dull or injured as it will enable you to learn to rely on one by itself. Cover your eyes and ears, and concentrate on just trying to use smell independently. Then cover your eyes and nose, and try to use your hearing alone. Finally, cover your nose and ears and use only your eyes.

Our senses, like the rest of our bodily functions, work best when used. Otherwise they will stagnate. Keep this in mind as you proceed.

Your Vision   You can exercise your visual ability by studying and closely observing colors, textures, shapes, shadows, and shading. Do this in landscapes, on flowers, trees and rocks.

Sweep a small area with your eyes and try to remember as many details about it as you can. Do this in a variety of situations like a park, a city street, inside a museum, or a store. Time yourself, by counting up to a certain number (say thirty), and then decreasing the time as you become more proficient.

Most of us let our line of sight direct our other senses. We begin to concentrate on what we are looking at, and the focus of our attention blots out other things around us. When we do this, we are no longer aware of all our surroundings, but only a very small segment of them, and this can be deadly. By keeping one's eyes moving, the senses also follow and remain active, and we remain safer.

We are also taught at a young age to restrict our visual field. This occurs when we are required to watch the blackboard, the teacher, and most of all, the TV screen. In fact, we continue it as adults, especially in this age of computers. And since our senses follow our line of sight, they too become diminished. This adversely affects our ability to discern human movement and spot an assailant lurking somewhere, or stalking someone. This is why learning to use peripheral vision becomes so important to our survival. In order to break the old habit of viewing the world as if through a tunnel, which by the time we reach adulthood has become automatic, we must learn to widen our visual field, as if everything before us was on a wide motion-picture screen.

One exercise Brown suggests is to look out into a landscape as you would normally. Then begin widening your vision by pretending the whole scene is a picture hanging on the wall. As you observe the entire landscape, push the frame as far out as you can.

Another technique is to stand with arms stretched out from your sides at right angles to your body, and wave your fingers. Look straight ahead and gradually expand your vision until your waving fingers come into view.

You can try other similar activities, depending upon your creativity. For instance, with your arms outstretched at right angles to your body, hold two small flashlights (they must be identical) in each hand. Turn

Retraining your eyesight can save your life by enabling you to isolate danger and focus on escape routes.

*Temporarily
eliminating one of
the senses
heightens the
remaining senses.*

them on and slowly move your arms towards each other until you can see the light, and then back again. To increase the challenge, you can use other objects with varying colors and brightness.

An outdoor activity requiring two people involves having someone walk a few yards behind you, holding a handful of white pebbles or beans. Every now and then the person should throw one to your left or right, or high over your head. As soon as you see it, point to it or call out. You will unconsciously begin to maintain a wider angle of vision for longer intervals from one toss to another, and it will soon become habit.

With practice, these exercises will help you to increase the scope of your peripheral field.

There is a natural phenomenon that occurs when people view a scene for the first time. We tend to fixate on its most obvious and distinctive features. The more we are familiar with these scenes, the more our line of vision returns to those same conspicuous features, and the more we neglect the unfamiliar, the less noticeable, and more obscure.

Try to look at your familiar surroundings as if each time is the first time you have seen them. This method helps to remove some of the automation that happens unconsciously.

Whether indoors or outdoors, for training to be effective all of these exercises should take place in varying lighting conditions.

Your Hearing Our auditory discrimination can also be trained. Listen to sounds that are mixed up with other sounds, such as those in music. Pick out the different instruments in a symphony orchestra.

Blindfold yourself in different surroundings and try to pick out and identify what you hear. Blindfolding also heightens and exaggerates other senses, making them more acute.

Listen to your surroundings from different distances and see if it makes a difference in your ability to trace what you hear and locate the source.

In social situations try tuning in to a conversation taking place away from you. See if you can make out any part of the conversation.

Cupping your hands around your ears can also help you to pick up sounds that would ordinarily be elusive.

There are also audio-training tapes available for this purpose. (*See Recommended Resources.*)

Your Sense of Smell Odor might be the only tell-tale sign that someone is lurking waiting to attack you. Being able to detect and discriminate odors is as important in the realm of survival as all your other senses.

To increase your ability to differentiate odors, blindfold yourself and have someone bring a variety of different-smelling objects and articles near you. The greater their variety, the better. Try using perfumes, foods, tobaccos, solvents, soaps, flowers, and the smell of different woods. Then have someone mix odors, first two together, then three, and try to identify each.

Practice separating and defining odors in your daily activities.

Detecting Danger with Your Senses

Here are a few examples of using your senses correctly to detect possible dangers.

Using Sight:

✔Catch a glimpse of someone moving close to you.

✔Notice a stranger staring at you, then turning away when you make eye contact.

✔Observe shadows.

✔Notice a burning cigarette on the ground ahead of you.

✔Notice the same person (or car) in your vicinity frequently.

✔See the sun reflect off a bright object ahead of you.

Using Sound:

✔Listen for human movement.

✔Hear a cough or sneeze, or clearing of the throat.

✔Hear a match being struck.

✔Hear a knife being opened.

✔Listen for any noise that seems out of context.

Intuition is a powerful tool, but is often disparaged in our highly intellectualized society.

> Walk with purpose, hold yourself with confidence: assailants read body language first.

Using Smell:

✔ Smell aftershave lotion.

✔ Smell pipe tobacco, cigar, or cigarette smoke.

✔ Smell body odor.

✔ Smell the lingering odor from a match being struck.

High-Level Intuitive Skills

Your intuition, gut feelings, or sixth sense is your best warning system. It is better than any radar. Operating together with your physical senses, it is unequaled in your arsenal of defense. If you pay attention to it always, it will neither let you down nor malfunction.

The best way to use your intuition is not to second-guess yourself, and if there is the slightest hint that it is telling you something, heed the message. Crime statistics are compiled in part from people who did not pay attention to their intuition.

That our intuition exists has been shown and accepted. It refers to the sum total of all our past experiences, some of which may have in some way registered in us, although unremembered, producing a special method of perceiving and evaluating objective reality.

One of the reasons that intuition is so crucial is that the number of our response/escape options decreases as an assault progresses. The earlier a potential victim can be alerted, the greater the chance of countermeasures succeeding.

In speaking to survivors over the years, I invariably ask them to try to remember if they had any inkling or hint before they were attacked. I rarely receive a negative response. Their reasons for not heeding their feelings are similar: They thought they were overreacting, they didn't want to act like a fool, or embarrass themselves, or seem paranoid. They added that they would never disregard their gut feelings again.

Formulating Your Strategies

You must learn to formulate strategies for when to talk, fight, and run. As the danger becomes more real, a number of possible responses will begin to surface. We must have a variety of effective response options readily available for situations of potential or real danger. How we match our response to the situation will depend upon the assailant's method of approach, and the stage which the assault has reached. How to formulate strategies can best be understood in relationship to the actual assault process.

Street assaults generally follow predictable patterns. An aggressive assault usually follows three distinct stages, which are closely related to the style of approach used by an assailant. These stages have been described by Joel Kirsch, a California psychologist and student of the martial art aikido, and author/psychologist/aikido master George Leonard who developed an assault-prevention course. Each stage is seen to have its own options for responses, and its opportunities for escape with minimal danger. They can be described as the invitation, confrontation, and altercation stages.

Invitation Stage   People do not purposely or consciously set themselves up to be attacked, but victims often unknowingly transmit their vulnerability. Muggers and rapists say it takes no more than ten seconds to size up potential victims based upon an analysis of their body movements. Assailants see vulnerability as opportunity and invite themselves into a situation. (See Chapter 4)

Confrontation Stage   At the very beginning of this stage, an important phenomenon comes into play as two people come close to each other. It is called the "holding mechanism," and it subconsciously draws our attention towards anyone who approaches us. An assailant has to "capture" and hold a potential victim's attention long enough to establish the respective roles each will take in the assault process—his role as "attacker" and the other's as "victim." The outcome of an assault often depends upon that split second when these roles are being defined. If you make a decision to resist, this is the best time to act on it. It shows the potential assailant that you are not yet defeated, and certainly do not identify yourself as a victim. It is during this stage that resistance stands the best chance of success.

Breaking the holding mechanism. Most assailants have their own plan of attack—what they expect as a result of each subsequent move. Their agenda may be based upon years of experience determining what will work "best."

Any unexpected variation introduced by a potential victim during

Surprise is an excellent form of defense.

Being prepared does not mean sticking to a pre-set plan regardless of the turn of events.

this stage can be a deterrent, causing the attack to be broken off and the assailant to wait for a more "suitable" victim. Coming up with something unanticipated that might produce concern or anxiety in the assailant and throw him off balance psychologically will often work. Your ability to do this effectively is part of your edge.

As an example, my son was performing at Lincoln Center, New York City. Wearing a tuxedo, he was walking during intermission to the men's room. The corridor was deserted except for a girl in a leather jacket, leaning against a corner—looking definitely out of place, and somewhat suspicious. Then, a male slowly began walking behind him, and out of the corner of his eye, my son noticed some fleeting recognition take place between these two people. He was now reasonably sure he was being set up for a mugging. He approached the men's room entrance, paused, looked inside, made a fast about-face, walked past his follower, smiled, and gave him a wave. Nothing happened. His would-be assailants were taken by surprise. By the time they had gathered their wits, it was all over. He had broken the holding pattern.

A method that has been used successfully by some potential victims is acting in a bizarre, irrational fashion, as if they were mentally disturbed. Many assailants would rather look for another victim than deal with this type of unpredictable behavior—especially if the assailant is a rapist. Several women have told me that this worked for them.

During this confrontation stage, you will either extricate yourself or convey nonverbally that you have been "captured." While this stage lasts only a few crucial moments, this is when the fear, panic, and paralysis may be produced which attackers rely on to turn people into victims.

Altercation Stage   If you reach this stage, it often involves facing a weapon. Most fatalities arise from guns, with knives coming in next. The general consensus of opinion from law enforcement people is that it is always best to cooperate with an assailant. This means giving him what he wants as quickly as possible. If he has a deadly weapon such as a knife or gun, resistance could lead to serious injury. Of course, there are situations where active resistance and being injured might be the better, more realistic choice. For instance, an assailant may clearly indicate that he intends to physically injure you. If your life appears to be in danger and you decide to use such countermeasures as running, distracting him, trying to attract attention or fighting, you must be alert to your assailant's behavior. If his guard drops, or if you see a clear opportunity to fight or run, you must then decide what to do. Anything that will save your life, curtail injury, and which you feel will work for you is the right thing to do.

On the other hand, your assailant may not indicate that he has a weapon at all, or he might threaten you with a concealed one, or have his hand in his pocket or under his coat as if he is holding one. In this situation you can either take his word for it, or ask to see it. Again, what your intuition tells you is very important.

If you face a weapon, do not let yourself be overwhelmed by it. For example, staring at it could induce more fear and terror in you, making it increasingly difficult to act decisively when you still have the chance.

The longer you can negotiate and buy some time, the more options become possible. However, should events get out of hand, you might find yourself completely at your attacker's mercy, with no options. If he wants to tie you up, lock you in a closet, take you in a car, or immobilize you in any way, you need to find ways you can refuse. (See Chapter 13)

You also have the option to do nothing. You may choose to use this approach until you can calm yourself enough to think straight, and decide what to do. Or you may choose to do nothing—period. Doing nothing at all is an option when you are sure that giving your assailant what he wants will result in your release unharmed. Or you may choose it if your actions might jeopardize the life of someone you are with, or if your assailant is holding you at gunpoint, or he is in a drug- or alcohol-induced state, or if you are outnumbered (see Chapter 13.) and have absolutely no options open to you. Drugs or alcohol can cause a person to become so out of control, impulsive, and unpredictable, that doing anything might be misinterpreted by him. Even when you choose to do nothing, this decision should never be absolute or final. You must remain aware, alert, and instantly ready to act if an opportunity presents itself.

You might try talking your way out of an assault by putting on an act (such as feigning illness), screaming, stalling for time, or using some means of distraction.

I remember a situation where, after robbing a series of stores, an attacker took a man hostage. He wanted to lock his hostage in the trunk

By continuously assessing the situation you will be prepared to change tactics in a split second.

of his car. The man pleaded with his assailant not to do it because he had claustrophobia and was successful in gaining his release.

It is impossible to predict the success of any negotiation because it depends upon several factors:

✔ *your assailant's personality, and how receptive he is to what he is hearing;*

✔ *what you are saying;*

✔ *your emotional tone and how convincing you sound.*

If you have actually extricated yourself with verbal means alone, stop talking and get away as soon as you have succeeded. You might just say that one more thing which could make your attacker change his mind. Get to safety as fast as possible.

When you have decided to run, you must feel confident that you can successfully meet these three conditions:

✔ *discover an available escape route;*

✔ *outrun your assailant;*

✔ *reach a place of safety.*

Failure in any one of these could be fatal. Once you decide to run you must keep on going until you reach safety. Do not stop to look around.

Fighting may become necessary if your life is on the line, and it is either you or him. In this case, you must fight to do as much harm to your attacker as you can, in any way you can, with no holds barred.

If you have succeeded in fighting off your assailant, do not relax your vigilance until you are sure you have reached safety. Remember, you have succeeded this far, and the worst is over. Keep yourself on the right track.

To summarize, in any assault situation the types of resistive strategies you choose will depend upon the following critical factors:

✔ *your emotional readiness to resist;*

✔ *the assailant's method of approach;*

✔*your degree of alertness and speed of reaction;*

✔*the stage to which the assault has progressed before you respond;*

✔*whether you feel your life is in imminent danger.*

The cardinal rule which always applies is that the situation itself should dictate your response.

Protective Devices

If you carry a protective device, be ready to use it at a split second's notice. Its use should be reflexive, instantaneous, and purposeful. (See Chapter 10 for objects that can be used in self-defense.)

Even if you never use any of the self-protective skills you have acquired, your self-assurance and the feeling that you are emotionally and physically capable of protecting yourself enhances your self-confidence and lessens feelings of vulnerability.

WHEN PUSH COMES TO SHOVE

Have you ever really stopped to think what you would do if you had to choose between defending yourself or possibly being killed if you did not? It is a frightening thought, but it is better to think about it in safety than when you are in harm's way.

Though secondary, you must consider the use of combative measures as a viable alternative when your life is actually on the line. This is when such measures may be your only recourse for survival. Defensive survival psychology points to the necessity of a potential victim being able to feel some degree of control in a dangerous situation, rather than feeling completely helpless. If you are to survive, you must psychologically as well as physically feel that part of your ability to survive is in your own hands. By ignoring the fact that combative measures may become necessary when faced with a choice between life or death, we lose sight of the important interaction between our physical and psychological experience. In summary, in order to maintain any hope of survival, we must never give up emotionally or physically, for if we do, it will decrease our strength before, during, and following the victimization.

Psychological preparedness includes feeling ready and able to defend yourself physically.

FACING LIFE-THREATENING ASSAULT: THE F.I.T. METHOD

Don't give an assailant the upper hand—be aware of your surroundings at all times.

As explained earlier, many factors occur simultaneously during any assault: those relating to the environment in which it is occurring, and the psychological and physical factors relating to victim and attacker. In order to survive in such a complex situation, we must be able to think straight and act decisively, despite the terrible anxiety we are feeling. No small task, indeed!

So what are we to do, and how are we to do it? We must be able to weed out what is and is not important in this survival process, and keep our sights on them. This is why a prescribed method involving specific steps must be adhered to. Remember, survival depends upon our minds and bodies working together.

This approach is not a mechanical one, or something to be memorized like a formula. In these pages we are going to learn to do many different things, and the process is a fluid one: all of our actions will combine and operate cohesively, some coming into play together, and some at different times.

Our Physical Behavior

In order to be aware of what is going on around us, we must first focus on it. Think of focusing a camera. When looking through the viewfinder you can't make out much of the features of the environment until they are sharply and clearly in focus. Similarly, when facing danger, if you merely glance around an area in a cursory manner you will be unprepared to take the next step. Instead, you must direct your attention in such a way as to allow you to separate out what does and does not belong—to isolate any signs that may indicate danger. The focusing (F.) and isolating (I.) stages are also extremely important because these stages are when intuitive feelings usually make themselves known. Whatever you decide to do, whether it is evasive or confrontational, you must be totally committed to carrying your course of action through to successful completion. In order to succeed, you must do it correctly. Your technique (T.) becomes crucial. Technique refers to the exact steps you intend to take; the quality of your actions, posture, timing, and all the things that will go into making them a success. In developing your technique, you must consider all possible contingencies. For instance, you may find that you have to make changes or substitutions before or during an attack, and this technique should be executed only when you feel that you have it down pat. If you act without a plan, the outcome could be deadly.

Our Emotional/Psychological Reactions

The way you are feeling will to a great degree influence which course of action you pursue. By feeling, I refer to psychological, not physical

The **F.I.T.** Method

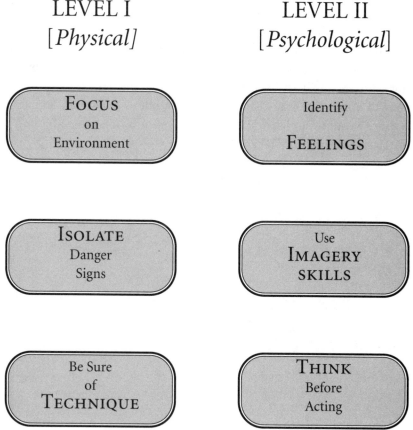

LEVEL I
[Physical]

LEVEL II
[Psychological]

FOCUS
on
Environment

Identify
FEELINGS

ISOLATE
Danger
Signs

Use
IMAGERY
SKILLS

Be Sure
of
TECHNIQUE

THINK
Before
Acting

Your thoughts and feelings will affect the outcome of an assault.

feelings (F.), because our physical capabilities can be either augmented or restricted by our mental state. How scared, confident, hesitant, reluctant, decisive, optimistic, angry, and so on are you feeling? Is it realistic to feel that your objective will be accomplished? One rape victim might be angry enough to fight off her attacker at all costs; another might be more scared and decide to give in to his demands; another might feel confident and decisive enough to try yet another approach. This assessment process might have to be done with such speed that you may question and second-guess your decisions. Don't worry. If you are able to do this under stress it means you still have your wits about you, and chances are you made the right decision initially. Without being impulsive, you should think (T.) before you act and choose the right moment to act decisively.

After you have made your choice, you are at the threshold for action. By now your imagery skills (I.) may have come into play, or you may be using them now for the first time. Imagery (discussed in Chapter 9) is the process of directing your mind to visualize something by using your imagination. You visualize the scenario step-by-step, from start to finish. The stage is set. Your technique is down pat, and your feelings about what you will be doing as you imagine yourself doing it are clear. You are ready for the final move.

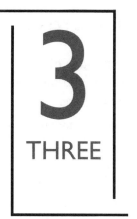

Why Me?

3

THREE

YOU CAN CONTROL the circumstances that lead to victimization by learning to alter possible risk-producing behavior, and by understanding how becoming a victim of crime may not always be just a matter of bad luck, or being in the wrong place at the wrong time.

ENVIRONMENTAL FACTORS

Environmental factors are related to one's lifestyle and everyday living habits, such as:

✔*Having a job requiring you to work late hours, in bad neighborhoods, or carry large sums of money and valuables. Many persons who have had to carry valuable gems as part of their job have been robbed or murdered.*

✔*People who are public figures, make their wealth evident, are very visible, adhere to a routine, or have predictable patterns of behavior. Numerous entertainers have been stalked, harassed, and murdered by so-called fans. Such people are easily found.*

✔*Being at the "right" place where an assailant happens to be looking for a victim. How many times have you heard the expression, being in the wrong place at the wrong time? Walking down a deserted street where an assailant is waiting, for example.*

PHYSICAL AND PSYCHOLOGICAL FACTORS

You can learn what factors lead to becoming a repeat victim of crime and thus prevent it from happening again.

There are many subtle cues we unknowingly convey through our feelings and behavior. These may become evident to others and increase our risk of being attacked or victimized. Among these cues are:

✔ *appearing to be a "safe" victim, who poses no threat of future retaliation against the assailant.*

✔ *appearing lax about our possessions, property, family, and ourselves;*

✔ *appearing to be less able to protect ourselves, like some women, children, the elderly, mentally handicapped, the emotionally disturbed, and physically disabled;*

✔ *unknowingly inducing anger, resentment, fear, embarrassment, or shame in others;*

THE TERRIBLE RISK TRIO:
FEELINGS OF GUILT, VULNERABILITY,
AND LACK OF CONFIDENCE

There is a very real relationship between feelings of guilt and vulnerability, and lack of confidence, since they are all involved in one way or other in our sense of well-being. The term well-being refers to a host of positive feelings about ourselves. Those of us who feel them are for the most part confident, self-assured, patient, in control, relaxed, secure, optimistic, and free of debilitating feelings of guilt and vulnerability. However, when we do not feel good about ourselves, a host of other feelings can prevent us from doing the very best we can. Lack of well-being can make us feel and act sluggish, confused, preoccupied, apathetic, restless, impatient, impulsive, pessimistic, depressed, jealous, irritable, moody, critical, tense, apprehensive, easily upset, hesitant, easily distracted, easily discouraged, inadequate, ill-at-ease, and generally unhappy.

Any or all of these feelings can increase our chances of becoming a victim, as we are more concerned with ourselves and less with what is going on around us. The positive feelings that go along with a state of well-being free us from these constraints, allowing us to stay alert, thereby decreasing our chances of becoming a victim.

A Feeling of Guilt

Guilt is a feeling of wrongdoing. It is also one aspect of fear, where what we fear is not immediately clear to us. It brings with it a feeling of anxiety, which is a fear of anticipated danger. Guilt arises from the part of our personality that judges, condemns, and criticizes. It brings a fear of being unmasked, of having our weaknesses revealed both to ourselves and to others. How we perceive these weaknesses is the result of our values. Guilt comes from our fear of punishment, and our sense of deserving it, rather than resulting from the punishment itself.

Some forms of proneness to victimization may result from unconscious guilt feelings that are felt to demand punishment. In such cases, if guilt feelings are aroused, this sense of deserved punishment may be followed by behavior that actually leads to punishment being suffered.

A Sense of Vulnerability

A sense of vulnerability is feeling that you are in the presence of either physical or emotional danger. A feeling of vulnerability can lead to indecisiveness, morbid fears, lack of assertiveness, fear of failure, inhibitions, lack of spontaneity, and the inability to think clearly and act purposefully in a critical situation.

A common symptom of vulnerability is the fear of retaliation from others, and always expecting the worst. Vulnerability can also make itself known in feelings of weakness, inferiority, inadequacy, and incapability. All of these may immobilize you in a life-threatening situation.

A Lack of Self-Confidence

Confidence is a feeling of trust and belief in our capabilities and the expectation that we will be successful.

A feeling of confidence is a key factor in our ability to deal effectively with everyday situations. Without such self-confidence, we develop feelings of inadequacy and a generally negative picture of ourselves. Our ability to be assertive and act aggressively is directly related to confi-

> *It is important to learn ways to decrease anxiety and feelings of vulnerability and guilt.*

It has been estimated that five out of six people will be victims of a violent assault at least once during their lives.

dence. We can take charge of a situation, life-threatening or not, only if we have sufficient self-confidence.

Dealing With Feelings of Guilt, Vulnerability, and Lack of Confidence

We have many ways to try to protect ourselves from these feelings. Here, I will consider those which can affect our physical well-being in a life-threatening situation. Some people try to be overly aggressive, putting on a facade of toughness or acting cocky in order to compensate for their lack of confidence and fear of failure. This can cause them to act impulsively and use poor judgment, putting their lives in jeopardy. Others may adopt a too-submissive and docile manner, shunning situations where assertiveness is necessary. Under certain circumstances, those who consistently deal with problems in this way also put their lives at risk. In these ways we may become victims of our own feelings of guilt, vulnerability, and lack of self-confidence, blocking our ability to cope effectively when faced with a victimizing experience.

Nothing can make you feel quite as guilty and vulnerable, and shatter your self-confidence, as becoming the victim of assault. The psychological impact coupled with bodily harm can produce a profound and long-lasting trauma, even for the most well-adjusted and problem-free individual.

This kind of trauma also has a way of arousing vivid feelings of guilt, vulnerability, and lack of confidence quite unrelated to the assault. These are feelings which often have been completely forgotten over the years, but surface again during psychotherapy.

For those who were victimized as children, guilt may develop and carry into their adult life over not having told someone. There may be guilt over the effects on their marriage, their social and sexual adjustment, or what they perceive was their role in causing parental discord, being "bad," doing something wrong, or being a disappointment to their parents.

Victims of crime may feel guilt over having been assaulted, over being selected as a victim, over not fighting back, or being unsuccessful in stopping an attack.

Victims of domestic violence may feel guilt over not being able to stand up to an abusive spouse, over their nonassertiveness both in and outside of the marriage, or over what they believe to have been their part in creating the problem.

For rape victims, guilt may emerge regarding what they believe to have been their role in attracting or provoking the rape, over having allowed it to continue, or over it happening at all.

Adults who were victims of child sexual abuse usually carry feelings of guilt over it happening to them, over what they perceive to have been their role in causing it to happen and in letting it continue, over not having told someone, and even guilt over the effects it has in their marriage or sexual adjustment.

Such guilt can have devastating effects on the survival process. For the body to function effectively, the mind must be free to allow it to do so.

PREVENTING CRIME

Rather than looking at what the individual can do, crime prevention discussions usually refer to the underlying social conditions producing it: alcohol, drugs, unemployment, poverty, and so on. And most people's attempts to do something preventative for themselves tend to be restricted to installing protective devices in their homes, not going out at night, and joining neighborhood watch programs. Few think in terms of doing something preventative on a more personal level. And few realize that even if the crime rate percentage points drop, the risk of violence and danger to each person remains relatively unchanged.

Studies have shown that only a very small percentage of people believe they are likely to become victims of crime; most feel that they are less likely than others to be victimized. This is what I have referred to as the "It can't happen to me" syndrome, described in Chapter 2. Anyone with this belief who becomes a victim must cope with both the direct consequences of the attack itself, and the loss of belief in their own invulnerability. While an illusion of invulnerability may protect us from the anxiety associated with the threat of all kinds of dangers, there are consequences to having such perceptions.

Crime prevention in most societies has primarily rested with the citizenry and not the police. The belief that we as individuals can pre-

For victims of assault and abuse, guilt can be profound and devastating.

> Approximately half
> of the population
> will be victims of
> violent crime more
> than once.

vent and survive a criminal attack is evident in the large amount of literature, films, public crime-prevention instruction, and self-defense courses devoted to techniques to reduce our chances of becoming victimized.

Crime Prevention and Self-Blame

Self-blame is classified into two categories: characterological and behavioral self-blame. The former is considered to be more related to our personality, making us see ourselves in a demeaning light. If someone like this is attacked, they are more likely to say such things as, "Everything happens to me," "It serves me right, I deserved what I got," "Everything I do is wrong." This kind of reaction is self-destructive, providing little confidence towards the prevention of future victimization.

Behavioral self-blame, on the other hand, is more constructive and has to do with the way in which we view our own behavior. If we are able to say, "I'm not going to let myself get into a predicament like that again," "I shouldn't have been walking there in the first place," or "I have to be more careful and aware from now on," then we are constructively looking for ways of preventing a repetition. Behavioral self-blame can be helpful in re-establishing a realistic sense of our vulnerability. It also helps us to prevent subsequent victimization via an underlying belief in our ability to exert some control over and thereby to modify possibly menacing future events.

BODY LANGUAGE: IT TELLS IT LIKE IT IS

There is mounting evidence that our feelings and attitudes directly influence our physical selves: how we move and breathe and even how we choose our physical and emotional experiences. Our behavior differs depending on our frame of mind. Our feelings are unconsciously conveyed to others and make themselves known in all kinds of unwitting behavior which may convey weakness, vulnerability, lack of confidence, and poor self-esteem. Among animals it is not accidental that the weakest of the herd is stalked by the predator. Likewise, human predators have their own stalking criteria.

In their classic 1981 study, professors Betty Grayson and Morris I. Stein demonstrated how body language was a contributing factor in attracting assailants. While walking in a high-assault area of New York City, people were videotaped at random for about seven seconds, the time it usually takes an assailant to size up a potential victim. They were unaware they were being taped. The tapes were evaluated at two different times by two different sets of prisoners who had been convicted of assault crimes.

Potential victims of an attack were seen to walk differently from most people. The study noted five basic characteristics of movement which distinguished victims from nonvictims.

✔ *Stride length: the distance between steps. The potential victims walked with exaggerated strides, extra long or extra short.*

✔ *Weight shift: the shift that occurs when transferring weight from one foot to the other while walking. Movement usually starts at the pelvis. The victims moved their bodies so that body weight would shift from side to side, diagonally, or with an up/down movement rather than in combination, as if their upper bodies moved at cross-purposes to their lower bodies, the halves appearing disconnected.*

✔ *Body movement: using one side of the body or one limb (unilateral movement) as contrasted with two sides of the body moving in counterpoint (contralateral movement). Potential victims moved unilaterally, one side at a time. They swung the arm and leg on the same side of the body simultaneously, rather than moving contralaterally (swinging the left arm together with the right leg and vice versa). Even those victims who moved contralaterally moved their upper and lower body parts against each other, rather than together.*

✔ *Type of walk: postural versus gestural movement, or how much the body participates in a movement. In postural movement, the initiation of movement comes from the center of the body, and is reflected in the total body moving as a coordinated unit, while gestural movement comes from the body's extremities and is limited to individual body parts. Potential victims walked gesturally, with their arm and leg movements appearing to come from their outer bodies rather than from within.*

> *Your demeanor and how you carry yourself can be like red flags to assailants.*

Violent crime
increased 260 %
from 1960 to
1975, and an
additional 84 %
from 1975 to
1991, according to
Uniform Crime
Reports.

✔Feet: *whether foot movement is swinging or lifted. Potential victims lifted and placed their whole foot at once as if walking on eggs rather than using a more fluid swinging heel-to-toe movement.*

The main difference between the two groups was described in terms of "wholeness" of movement. The body parts of potential victims seemed to be working against each other, giving the impression that the body was not moving as a total unit. In contrast, the movements of those who were not rated as potential victims were more unified and originated from the body's center. In addition, walking with a fixed gaze up or down suggests preoccupation, and a distinctly slower stride than other foot traffic attracts attention.

Body Language from a Scientific Perspective

Dr. Ida Rolf, a well-known biochemist and physiologist, studied the body's response to different mental states. She noted that both physical and emotional traumas cause our muscular and facial tissues to become tight and rigid. The body then tends to move from a state of natural alignment and vitality towards overall inflexibility and gravitational imbalance. This continuing condition in turn may limit our range of emotional flexibility. She observed that when someone experiences temporary fear, grief, or anger, their body is often carried in such a way that the particular emotion is recognizable by others. If this condition persists, or is consistently repeated, a physical habit pattern is formed and the body's muscular arrangement becomes set. The person assumes an involuntarily restricted physical demeanor which in turn actually leads to the establishment of a more limited and restricted emotional pattern.

We have all experienced how eye contact is usually the first communication between two people; it is, therefore, very important. Any time one person meets the gaze of another, each receives a whole series of impressions. These "messages" play a prominent role in how each will behave towards the other.

Think, for example, of how you look at others, and how some people look at you. Think of how you feel when one stranger stares at you with a piercing look, and another refuses to meet your gaze, immediately dropping his or her eyes to the ground. Each of these people is conveying feelings, and in turn evoking yours. The manner in which you handle eye contact could be the deciding factor in your becoming a victim, whether you are walking on the street, riding a bus, or in a museum. For instance, staring a person into oblivion could label you as someone looking for trouble, and elicit an aggressive response from a potential assailant. On the other hand, refusing to look at someone at all could convey feelings of fear and vulnerability.

Sexual assault research suggests that women who have been taught the traditional feminine nonaggressive role convey cues in their appearance which hint that they are vulnerable to aggression. This role is usually developed when as little girls they are encouraged to express passivity, dependency, and submissiveness through their physical appearance.

Body Language and Environmental Conditions

There are other factors which also have a bearing upon our body language. We see them before us every day, adjust to them in numerous ways, take them for granted, and do not give a second thought to their significance for our survival. They are the climate, weather, lighting conditions, and time of day, and each has a unique way of affecting our appearance and manner. They influence the types of clothing we wear which, in turn, affects our freedom of movement and our walking habits. The heavier, more bulky, or longer the clothing, the more it will modify our way of walking as well as making it more difficult to fight or run.

Weather and climatic conditions can also affect our mood, alertness, and behavior. People often feel more gloomy in bad or rainy weather than in nice weather. A gloomy feeling can prevent you from functioning at optimal levels, and make you less vigilant. On the other hand, a bright sunny day might lead you to feel happy, cheerful, or carefree, and to walk around with your head in the clouds—a state of mind which could also make you less alert and watchful.

During cold weather you may think more about keeping warm; hot weather might cause you to become sluggish. Either may decrease your awareness. Wet or slippery streets not only decrease your agility and mobility, but divert your attention away from the rest of your surroundings. You may be concentrating more on keeping your footing, and less on your surroundings.

Eye contact, particularly between men and women, is read differently in different cultures.

Vulnerability can be tied to such factors as the weather and, in turn, the clothing we wear.

As dusk approaches, your visual acuity is cut down, as it is during cloudy, rainy, or snowy weather.

But remember that any increase in risk is directly related to how preoccupied you are and how much your guard is down at a given moment. The cause itself is unimportant. If you are less alert, you will be more vulnerable and this will be evident in your behavior for the wrong person to observe. But if you are alert and confident, it will show in your demeanor, and you will be ready to take the kind of preventive and defensive actions described in the following chapters.

4

FOUR

Reducing Your Risk

BEWARE BY BEING AWARE

AFTER READING THIS vast array of precautionary measures against becoming victimized, you might begin to imagine yourself in danger from the time you open your eyes in the morning to the time you close them at night. This chapter is not intended to induce a mental state of siege. But you should be prepared at all times. Why? Because your everyday crook, your everyday mugger doesn't give a hoot what he does or to whom he does it. He will take advantage of whatever opportunity turns up, whether it means knocking over a small elderly person for a few dollars, breaking into your house or car, or following you out of a building or store. And you must maintain appropriate balance and perspective, picking and choosing what applies to you and what does not and doing so without becoming paranoid.

THINGS TO KEEP IN MIND

✔ *Keep in mind that you should not expect to be able to identify a potential attacker from his appearance. Some of the most vicious and dangerous assailants can look no more threatening or different than your own son, brother, husband, or father.*

✔ *Keep in mind that your best defense is to outwit your assailant, not to outrun or outfight him. Remember, he has probably done this before and you haven't. The master key which can unlock all doors to survival is your own creativity.*

✔*Never—I repeat—never believe what your assailant tells you! What he says may be said to string you along, to keep you off guard, or your fears at a high level, or to get you to do what he wants with a minimum of resistance. It may all be a ploy to distract you from your immediate goal—which is escape. If you fall for any one of them, he will have accomplished his goal.*

While violent crime attracts a lot of media and public attention, it actually makes up only about 10% of all crime.

YOUR DAILY HABITS

The most important goal of risk reduction is to eliminate potentially threatening situations. Make this a daily habit.

Before you venture out onto the street, make preparations to ensure your safety. Wherever you are going plan the route you will take, letting someone know your approximate time of arrival. Check in by telephone with that person at a prearranged time. Be sure you always have enough change for a telephone, but leave unneeded credit cards, large amounts of money, or blank checks at home.

Plan ahead for unforeseen contingencies. Think of the worst things that could possibly happen along the way, for instance, if your car breaks down, or your purse is snatched, or you are being followed, and have some clear procedures ready to follow.

The following precautions take very little effort and have wide implications.

✔*Walk with a purpose, at a steady pace, back straight, head erect, and appear as if you know where you are going. Move from your center with a balanced stride. Do not become fixed on individual objects, but look around, and stay aware of your environment. Concentrating on too many specific things can cause you to lose touch with the street around you. Lightly swing your arms in a relaxed fashion to convey strength and confidence. Do not hold your hands in your pockets or close to your body as this will interfere with the wholeness of movement you must strive for.*

✔*It is best not to overdo eye contact in any way. When coming face to face with a stranger, let your eyes briefly meet his in an acknowledgement, and then continue about your business. There may be times when you want to add a brief smile, or a nod. This could psychologically disarm a potential assailant as it conveys a lack of fear, two things that assailants try to avoid in victims. They would rather see someone whose eyes are glued to the pavement. (If you recall, this is what my son did to break the holding mechanism in the incident at Lincoln Center in New York.)*

✔*Vary the routines of what you do and how you do it: the routes you follow, the transportation you use, the time schedules to which you adhere. Nothing increases risk more than a rigid lifestyle with highly predictable behavior patterns.*

✔*Whenever possible, shop during the day. The dark greatly increases the risk of an assault. When you leave a shopping area stay near a group of people rather than walking out alone, even if you have to wait a few minutes for people to appear.*

✔*It is always safer to go somewhere with a companion, whether it be to a movie, shopping, a restaurant, museum, jogging, bicycling, or just plain walking.*

✔*The less strangers know about you the better. If you are unmarried, do not advertise it by putting your name on the mailbox or in the telephone directory. Use initials. Do not give your address or telephone number to anyone without checking the person's credibility first.*

✔*If you are placing an ad in the paper, if possible do not use your home phone number. Use a business number.*

✔*If someone phones you by mistake, do not reveal your name or telephone number.*

✔*Be careful what is revealed by the message on your answering machine. It should say something like, "You have reached the Jones' residence. Please leave your message at the tone."*

✔*Never answer personal information questions over the phone to anyone you don't know. If the person claims to be conducting a survey, ask for something to be sent through the mail. If a sales representative wants to know if you own a certain product, do not give out any information.*

Dress "down" in public places. Keep flashy jewelry—real or costume—out of sight.

According to U.S. statistics the highest number of violent victimizations occur in the area where the victims live.

Ask what the call is about, and request that information be sent to you, or simply say you are not interested.

✔Crank telephone calls of the sort where someone offers information about you of a personal nature—your appearance, where you work, your habits, or things about your lifestyle—indicate that your caller has been studying you. Do not ignore this type of call, but report it to the police.

✔No matter where you might be, whether in a supermarket, beauty parlor, or museum, be careful how you speak to others about your personal life, travel plans, and general day-to-day activities. You never know who might be listening, and who they are.

REDUCING YOUR RISK IN YOUR HOME

✔If you are expecting someone, and might not be home, never leave a note on the door stating when you will return. It would give a robber time to break in and go through the house knowing he will not be interrupted.

✔Before letting a stranger into your house, ask for identification. This holds true for servicemen, meter readers, delivery people, or anyone with whom you are not personally familiar. Check them out by telephoning their company. If they have something that requires your signature, have them slip it under the door or leave it in the mailbox.

✔Never rely on a door's chain guard alone. Unless it is a special heavy-duty door, a strong person could rip the unit off wherever it is secured by throwing their weight against the door.

✔Wherever you are, if you sense potential danger, pretend that you are not alone. Convey to anyone listening or watching that you are expecting someone and that he or she is close by. If your doorbell rings and you are suspicious of the person, call to a make-believe husband in the next room loud enough for your caller to hear "Honey, can you get the door? I'm in the middle of cleaning the oven." Chances are any intruder will make tracks fast. If he persists, say through the closed door, "I can't open the door now and my husband is busy. Just leave your card under the door or in the mailbox." Or yell, "Harry, can you get the door?"

✔The next step is to call the police. In this situation do not ask your caller for a phone number to call for verification as it could be the number of an accomplice. If you do not answer the doorbell because of your suspicions, he could assume no one is home and proceed to break in. It is, therefore, advisable to yell loud enough to your make-believe person so your voice will carry through the door. Keep a variety of excuses in mind to be used in various situations. Remember, they have to be realistic, appropriate, and convincing.

✔Be suspicious of anyone at your door asking to use the telephone, or saying that their car has broken down. (Sometimes a woman will make the initial contact and have a male accomplice standing nearby out of view.)

✔Your home may be your castle, but it surely is not your fortress. Should you ever find yourself alone in the house with an assailant be prepared with two survival plans. The first and best one is to get out of the house. I am sure you have an escape route set up in case of a fire. You might want to follow this procedure, or adapt it with some changes.

✔The second plan is for what to do if you cannot get out. Crime prevention experts talk about setting aside a "safe room" where you can go to be protected from harm. This can be almost any room with a strong solid door, an inside lock, and a phone. A portable phone is ideal, in case your attacker cuts the phone wires. (A portable phone is always good to have, since it can go wherever you do.)

✔If you are asleep and are awakened by an intruder entering your home, do not let him know you are awake. Either play 'possum until he leaves, or wait for the right opportunity to make your way out of the house, to another part of it, or to summon help. If you try to escape, do so very slowly and quietly.

REDUCING YOUR RISK AWAY FROM HOME

✔Many assailants have injured or even killed a victim because they could not get enough money to satisfy themselves. Carrying extra money (sometimes called "mugger's money") on your person and also having some available at home could possibly save your life.

> Make a plan, think it through, act it out. Survival depends upon being mentally and physically prepared.

If you've got it, don't flaunt it. Flashing money and jewels is inviting danger.

✔*Take care when exposing money, no matter where you are—in a store, bank, building, car, or on the street. Muggers are always on the watch for people who advertise what they are carrying. When you receive change in folding currency, immediately put it into your purse or pocket, without opening your wallet and exposing more money. Never walk out of a store, bank, or other building counting or folding money. Not only are you putting it on display, but you are also not concentrating on your surroundings as you should be doing. Never leave loose money next to you on the seat of a car.*

✔*When shopping in a center or mall it is natural to be preoccupied, and to let down one's guard. Assailants watch for vulnerable targets in these situations. So be alert.*

✔*Assailants have been known to observe people carrying out transactions in a bank. A would-be mugger can stand watching outside, or even use binoculars from a car. It is always good practice to keep blank withdrawal slips at home so you can bring one already filled out to the bank. In this way, if you immediately walk up to the teller upon entering the bank, it will give the impression that you are making a deposit. Ask the teller to put the money in an envelope before she hands it to you, and then put it right into your pocket or purse before you leave the window. If you have to count it again, go to an area where no one can see what you are doing from the outside, and face the rear of the bank.*

✔*When you are in a bank, always stay alert as to who is around you. If you think you are being watched, let a teller or the manager know. And ask for someone to accompany you out of the bank.*

✔*Be extra alert when using automatic bank machines. This is a favorite place for muggers. If possible, have someone accompany you. As you approach, scan the area carefully. If you feel any uneasiness, do not proceed. Do not face the machine. Angle yourself so you can see what is going on around you while making your transaction. Put the money directly into your pocket or purse and leave rapidly. Do not count it or put it into a wallet until you are in a safe place.*

✔*You should learn to routinely stand and walk at an angle, and get into the habit of doing this no matter where you are. Instead of walking with* your body facing frontwards and both feet pointing ahead, try walking straight, then turn your body about forty-five degrees in one direction. You can avoid any tendency to veer off in that direction by making sure one foot always faces frontwards. For example, if you are angling your body to the left, make sure your right foot keeps going straight. Reverse the process for angling towards the right.

You will find that when you develop this habit, your awareness will increase by leaps and bounds. For instance, you should walk partially sideways for a few steps when entering or leaving an apartment, elevator, office, corridor, any building, car, or public conveyance. Angle yourself when standing to unlock your car, mailbox, and apartment door. Angle yourself when waiting for a bus, taxi, train, or to cross a street.

Angling yourself not only allows you to see what is behind you, but also indicates to an assailant that you are not going to be an easy target.

✔If you are in a strange area or lost, and you need assistance, do not stop just anyone to ask. Seek out a policeman, mailman, someone in a delivery truck, a storekeeper, or a service station attendant. Assailants looking for prey will easily spot someone in trouble.

✔When alone, stay out of stores late at night.

✔Do not go alone to public lavatories in restaurants, theatres, transportation terminals, or shopping centers. If you absolutely must go, try to let a friend know beforehand. Do not go all the way in unless there are already several people inside.

✔Never hitchhike and never pick up anyone on the road should be another rule of thumb. It could be a "fatal attraction."

✔Do not focus on appearances. Some assailants—like street-gang kids— may dress to frighten. They rely on the leather, chains, and other grotesque items to set off your fear reaction. Once they have accomplished this, they are on their way to success. Remember the mind's influence on the body, the fight-or-flight response, and how the body "freezes" when panic takes over? Well, do not forget that underneath the leather is a vulnerable body of skin and bones, and within the attacker's brain there is the same potential for intimidation and fear as there is in your own.

Robbery is the primary motive in almost half of violent crimes.

The 1990 juvenile arrest rate was 27% higher than in 1980.

✔*Avoid distractions whenever possible. A distraction can throw you off guard long enough to make you a victim. For example, bypass strange noises that might otherwise cause you to stop and investigate. This could be a ploy.*

✔*In a family, all members should have a prearranged method of communication in response to danger. In the event someone is unable to speak freely they can use agreed-upon verbal signals like a code.*

✔*Be alert to anything out of the ordinary that occurs in your life and in your environment that your intuition makes you question.*

Whenever you come into close proximity with a stranger there is a natural tendency for each of you to keep a certain distance, even where there is no feeling of threat. I call this keeping your psychosocial space. It is a good idea to maintain this psychosocial space in everyday life

✔*When walking do not allow your space to be invaded. If someone is coming directly towards you, veer away from him so as to maintain your own safe area. By making this a habit, you will accomplish three things.*

✔*Force a would-be assailant to make his intentions more obvious. The earlier you know whether you are in real danger or not, the faster you can act evasively.*

✔*Make it much more difficult, if not impossible, for the holding mechanism to operate (where an assailant feels he "has you," and you feel "in his clutches" before an actual confrontation).*

✔*Enable you to evade a potential attack much earlier, thereby giving you a chance to escape.*

More specific safeguards follow, relating to routine activities taking place on foot, in a car, involving public transportation, and when traveling away from home.

When You Are Walking

✔*Whether on the street or in parking areas, walk several feet away from parked cars, especially from vans with sliding doors.*

✔Similarly, keep away from buildings, shrubbery, doorways, stairwells, alleys, or dimly lit areas. This is especially important when approaching a corner. An attacker could be waiting just around that bend, and grab you as you pass.

✔Walk on the side of the street that faces oncoming traffic, no matter where you are going. In this way you will be alert to a driver or passenger of a passing car who may try to grab you. There is minimal risk of abduction from a moving car, although it has occurred, especially to women in sexual assault situations. Much more frequent is someone riding by and grabbing an easily accessible purse from a pedestrian.

✔Do not enter a tunnel or corridor before first checking the area to see if it is safe. Even if it appears safe inside, you do not know what will greet you on the other side. It is always best to avoid these places, if possible. If not, waiting for others to walk with you is the next best alternative.

✔Use the reflections in store windows as your own security mirror to see what is happening behind you or across the street.

✔If you are being followed on a well-traveled street, slow down, speed up, then reverse your direction to let your pursuer know you are aware of him. Then immediately seek help.

✔If you are being followed on a deserted street, get to a well-lighted and populated area as fast as possible. But do not run straight for home unless you know help will be readily available there.

✔If you are being followed by a car, reverse your direction, and try to find a store to enter, or a busy area.

✔Be aware of ways to attract attention. If there is a store with people in it that you can enter, do it. If you can flag a taxi or, if you must, even get into a car that is stopped for a light, do it. Or wave your arms to signal to motorists that you need help.

✔On busy streets, carry your purse or briefcase on the side farthest from the curb. If you are carrying a shoulder-strap purse or briefcase, it should hang straight down from your shoulder, held tightly between

When walking and jogging, never turn your back on potential danger: always face oncoming traffic.

Studies have found that those who take the fewest precautionary measures are more likely to be affected by crime.

your arm and body, with the flap facing in. Do not let it swing to and fro. If you are wearing a loose garment, like a jacket, coat, or outside shirt, let your bag hang underneath the garment.

✔ If you carry it exposed, never let a strap cross your body. If a thief were to grab the bag by this strap, you could be knocked down and dragged. Carry bags with short straps like a football, with the arm placed through the straps. When approaching anyone who looks suspicious, tighten your grip on whatever you are carrying. But wrapping the loop of any bag around your wrist will only cause you to be dragged to the ground if someone were to try to pull it from you. Try switching your handbag to an upside-down position, holding it closed with your hand. If someone tries to snatch it, the contents will fall to the ground, giving you a chance to run.

By far the safest way to carry your belongings is in the kind of purse that goes around your waist with a strap or belt. These are found in most luggage, sporting goods, and department stores.

✔ Try to see ahead of you as far as possible.

✔ Avoid using stairs whenever possible. They are a favorite area for muggers and rapists to hide and wait.

✔ When leaving work, or leaving a building with its own parking area, it is safer to walk in a group or with someone else.

✔ Use a public telephone only if it is in a well-populated area. As phoning is likely to preoccupy and distract you, try to be especially aware of what is going on near you. Never talk facing the phone. If you are in a booth with doors, try to keep them open for a fast exit if needed. At the first sign of danger, drop the phone and get away fast.

✔ If for any reason you must be in a public building after hours, on a weekend, or on a holiday, always have someone accompany you to the room you are going to, and make sure you are secure while there. When you leave also have your companion accompany you from your office to your destination.

✔ One of the best ways to attract attention if you find yourself in danger is to throw something through the front display window of a store or of-

fice—if you are fortunate enough to be near one. Nothing gets people's attention as fast as shattering glass. Chances are that your assailant will not be interested in remaining on the scene very long after this happens.

✔ *If you are on an escalator in a building and happen to see that there is danger on the approaching landing, do not hesitate. Whatever direction you are going, whether up or down, immediately turn around and retreat in the opposite direction, and try to go where there are other people.*

When You Are Jogging

✔ Never jog while listening to a radio or tapes through headphones, as you will not be able to hear suspicious sounds, such as someone stalking you nearby. And it will also decrease your general awareness and concentration so you will not be paying proper attention to your surroundings.

✔ It is advisable to always jog during daylight in populated areas, and with a partner.

✔ The more you vary your route, the better.

✔ Make note of avenues of escape or places where help might be available if it becomes necessary. Also make note of where the most dangerous or vulnerable areas for attack could be, and where someone could hide.

✔ If the route is familiar, be keenly aware of the danger signs of something being different, or of new people jogging near you.

✔ Pace yourself to maintain your stamina in case you have to quickly get out of the way of someone who is getting too close, or if you are getting too close to a runner who is a stranger.

✔ As in walking, keep a safe distance from buildings, alleyways, bushes, or questionable areas.

✔ Run against oncoming traffic, and in the opposite direction on one-way streets, so that no car can pull up alongside you.

Routine is the ally of the assailant: vary the times and locations of your activities.

Loud, piercing noises can startle and irritate: carry a whistle or personal alarm when out for a walk or jog.

✔Be aware of anyone coming up behind you. Change or reverse your direction. If the person follows you, change again, and this time try to find a safe haven or attract someone's attention. Use the same evasive tactics as those applied to walking, above.

✔If you run on a track, changing your direction from time to time will make it obvious if someone is following you.

✔It is a good idea to wear a loud whistle around your neck, or carry an alarm, in the event you need to attract attention.

✔As in all public activities, use all your senses to remain as aware of your surroundings as possible.

When You Are Cycling

✔The rules for joggers also apply to those on bicycles. When cycling keep on going and do not stop for anyone. It could be a ploy to get you to stop.

If a Stranger Stops You to Ask for Directions or the Time

✔Do not stand close to the person. Back away and slowly circle to one side to see if someone is behind you, or if there is an accomplice nearby.

✔Do not let yourself be in a position where you can be dragged into the car. If there is more than one person in the car, be even more cautious. It is best not to stop at all, and say "I'm sorry, but I'm late."

✔Check around you to see if someone is lurking nearby who could push you into a car, and be prepared to prevent this.

When You Are Approaching Your Home

✔Make sure there is nothing suspicious on the route you are taking.

✔If there is anyone who does not look right to you for any reason, do not continue onward. Alter your direction until this person has gone or you can find someone to accompany you home.

When You Are Entering an Apartment Lobby

✔ Before entering, check to see if anyone is in the lobby. If there is and you know no one is in your apartment, press the buzzer and wait. When there is no response, turn around and walk away. If, however, you know someone is home, do not press the buzzer, for if there is a response you will have to proceed inside. The clever thing to do is completely cover the button with your thumb but do not press it. It will be impossible for anyone to know whether or not you are exerting pressure.

✔ If you are being followed, pretend you are a visitor pressing the buzzer. Then leave.

✔ If a stranger is admitted as a visitor, do not follow him in. This does not mean he has passed inspection. Some people keep ringing bells until someone lets them in. Be alert to this. If he goes into the elevator, do not enter the building. He may be waiting for you.

When You Are Entering Your Apartment/House

✔ Make sure everything looks in order. If not, but everything is quiet, leave immediately. Go to a neighbor's and call the police.

✔ Upon confronting an intruder, do nothing to threaten him. He may be just as interested in getting away from you as you are in getting away from him. He may, therefore, leave faster than you. If not, try to get out yourself.

When You Are Waiting For an Elevator

✔ Stand well back and to the side of the doors and angle yourself so you cannot be pulled inside or pushed in from behind.

✔ If there is a stranger inside, do not enter.

✔ If the elevator you are in alone stops at a floor and a stranger gets in, immediately walk out at the same time. If you hesitate and the door begins to close, immediately press the "door open" or "door hold" button and leave.

> Do not enter your home if you suspect there is an intruder present.

> Property crime represents about half of all reported crime.

✔Inside an elevator always stand close to the control panel and angle yourself.

✔As an added precaution, press two or three extra buttons when you enter an elevator. This prevents another passenger from knowing where you are going, and also gives you an opportunity to get off earlier if necessary.

✔Always make sure the elevator is going in the direction you want to go before entering it.

✔If you are followed off an elevator, go to a few apartments or offices and ring their doorbells for help. The chances are that someone will be available in one of them.

✔Be suspicious if your elevator is out of service. Many assailants cause this to happen, and then wait for their victim by the stairwells. If this happens to you, call the superintendent or manager of the building before taking the stairs.

If You Are Attacked in an Elevator

✔Never press or allow your assailant to hold down the red emergency or stop button. This stops the elevator and you then become a captive. You can prevent this from happening by pressing as many buttons as possible, so that the elevator will continually stop at different floors. This will give you added opportunities to escape. Someone might even be waiting on one of the floors who will help you.

When You Are Walking to Your Car

✔If possible, walk to your car with someone, and then drive them to their car. Before driving off, arrange a signal indicating that everything is all right with each of you, such as a tap of the horn, or headlights going off and on. If this does not happen, follow the car, keeping a safe distance behind until you can find a police officer or other help.

✔Do not walk close to or between parked cars or obstacles behind which an assailant could be hiding. It is safest to walk in the wide traffic lanes.

✔ *Make sure no one is following you.*

✔ *Be suspicious if you see any unusual activity in the vicinity.*

When You Are Approaching Your Car

✔ *If there are people loitering nearby, go back and find someone to walk there with you.*

✔ *Look under your car, as well as under others close by. Do this from a distance as you are walking towards it. Walk around it, from the back to the front. If you are in a mall, with other cars parked next to, in front of, or in back of yours, stay a distance of about two car widths away and view the underneath at an oblique angle. In this way, as you circle the car, you will be able to see overlapping areas. An assailant may lie in wait under the car, to grab or slash your ankles as you are unlocking or opening the door.*

✔ *Check to see if the car appears to have been tampered with in any way and will not be able to move. Do not stand there if this is the case. Leave quickly to get help.*

✔ *Look at your car's tires, hood, trunk, doors, and windows for new scratches or tool marks, or dirt or grease that wasn't there before. Make sure there are no nails or broken glass around your car that could damage the tires.*

✔ *Make use of your windows' reflections. In certain lighting conditions, the glass will act as a mirror and reflect what is behind you.*

✔ *The speed with which you unlock and enter your car is important. With keys always ready in your hand, first angle yourself so you can see anyone coming from behind. Also check the back seat and floor before unlocking the door. This, of course, depends upon lighting conditions. Even at night, your car may be near a street light, or in an area where you can see inside. Carrying a small flashlight with you at night is a good idea. If everything is clear, unlock the door with one hand, and as you retract the key from the lock pull the door handle open with the other hand. These few seconds could be crucial in an assault situation.*

Because people tend to view their car as a safety zone, they often relax their vigilance when approaching it.

Invest in a small flashlight that can be attached to your keychain.

✔ Once inside the car immediately lock all doors.

✔ If something about the car doesn't feel right, but the car is operable, drive away and get it checked later on.

✔ If the car was OK before but now will not start, be suspicious. Do not accept any offers of assistance. Get out, lift the hood, get back in, and lock all doors. Try to get someone to call the police by opening your front window to ask for help—but open it only just enough to allow the person to hear you.

✔ Be wary of a van parked next to your car.

✔ Be wary of anyone sitting in a car parked next to yours.

✔ As in all enclosed areas, be aware of all elevators, stairwells, and passageways where an assailant could be hiding, as well as entrances and exits that could be used for escape routes.

When You Are Inside a Car

✔ Unless you are on a highway, keep doors locked and windows closed.

✔ When driving, be aware of what is going on ahead of and behind you.

✔ If you can take a longer route rather than going through a high-risk area, you should do so.

✔ Do not flash large amounts of money when paying tolls.

✔ Do not keep valuables in full view. The best place to keep bags or small cases is in the trunk, or on the floor of the car, close to the seat, with someone's legs covering them. If the items are too large, lay them flat on the floor with your legs stretched over them.

✔ If you are a woman driving alone at night, wearing a man's hat will disguise your sex. You can arrange pillows with a coat and hat over them to make it look like someone is sleeping in a passenger seat.

✔ If you have to stop and ask directions, open your window just enough to be heard.

✔When getting gas, do not give the attendant your other keys along with your gas-cap key, even for a moment. It takes no longer than that to take an impression of any key on the ring.

✔Keep at least a car's length behind the car in front of you so you can get clear in an emergency.

✔If, when you are stopped, someone approaches you and motions you to open the window, do not do so.

✔If you are signalled to stop by an unmarked car with a flashing light, or by someone who flashes a badge, or someone in uniform, never get out of your car. Keep the windows open just enough to ask for ID, which should include a picture. Not until you are absolutely certain everything is on the up and up should you do any more. Any true police officer can easily radio for a marked police car to arrive.

✔Do not pull off or stop on the road if someone is stalled in a car, lying on the road, or motioning to you for help. This can be a ploy. Report it to the first police officer you can find, or if you have a car phone, use it.

✔If someone tries to forcibly enter your car while you are stopped for a light, sound your horn and start moving even if you have to run a red light.

✔With the rising number of assualts occurring in garages, extreme caution must be taken when driving into one. While it is natural for a driver to be preoccupied with the door as it is opening, this decreases his or her awareness of the immediate surroundings. Stop the car and wait for the door to fully open. Focus on the surrounding area. When the door has stopped and if everything is clear, pull in. Watch through the rear-view mirror to make sure nobody enters while the door is closing. If the garage door operates manually, you do not have the added protection of remaining in a locked car. Before leaving your vehicle it is essential that everything looks normal. If there are any areas where an assailant could be hiding, such as shrubbery, a blind corner, or any obstruction, these should be scrutinized with extreme care. If you are not sure, do not pull in. Drive to a neighbor's house and either call the police or have the neighbor follow you back to your house in their car.

In any given year, there will be approximately six million people raped, robbed or assaulted in the U. S., and an estimated 21,000 murdered.

When You Are Parking

Always back into a parking space; you may need to leave in a hurry.

✔Try to select a public parking garage where you will not have to walk through a secluded area.

✔Leave only the ignition key with an attendant.

✔Take all valuables, garage door openers, and anything that can identify you or your residence out of the car.

✔When asked how long you will be gone, do not give a definite time, but make it relatively short. This way your car is likely to be kept in a more accessible space.

✔In a public parking area, do not park your car on the outer edges, where it is more likely to be tampered with, and where it is also more isolated for you to walk.

✔Try to point your car so that it will be easy to drive away in a hurry, even if you have to park it facing opposite to those next to you.

✔If possible, do not park next to a wall, ledge, column or similar structure, so that you cannot be trapped in this space when entering or leaving your car.

✔Never park next to a van. Assailants can be concealed in a van because many have no side windows. Their sliding side doors are easy to exit from and for pulling someone inside. It only takes seconds to grab you and pull you inside as you approach your car. If there was no van next to your car when you parked but now there is, do not walk to your car alone.

✔Never leave anything on the seats or dash while your car is unattended—not even an empty paper bag or some loose change. A thief on the prowl will not discriminate, but will break into a car if there is a possibility that something there may be of value.

If Your Car Breaks Down in a High-Risk Area

✔Open your hood and return to your car.

✔Lock all the car doors.

✔Do not accept assistance from any stranger.

✔Open your window just enough to ask someone to call the police.

If Your Car is Followed or Bumped from Behind

✔It is always best to keep behind someone who is out for trouble. Try to maneuver yourself into this position.

✔Try to get to a well-lighted, populated area where there might be stores and other traffic.

✔Pull into a service station or a police station.

✔Attract attention by slowing down, continuously sounding your horn, flashing your high beams, and putting on your rear hazard lights. Even go through traffic lights, if you must.

✔Try to find a police car, and cut it off if necessary.

DO NOT:

✔Allow yourself to panic.

✔Pull off to the side of the road to see if the car will pass you or what he will do next.

✔Go home (and reveal where you live).

✔Speed up if he is bumping you. He may continue bumping you, and at low speeds a car can sustain more abuse with less damage, and the driver can remain more in control. At high speeds the driver is less able to control his car and there is always maximum risk.

If You Are in a Car Accident

✔Assailants will sometimes deliberately cause an accident in order to get a victim.

> To escape assault, don't be afraid to break traffic rules.

> Courtrooms are backlogged. Prosecutors and judges make and accept plea bargains with even serious, violent offenders.

✔ *If you are involved in an accident, or if someone bumps you from behind, no matter where it happens, you are legally obliged to stop. But never get out of the car.*

✔ *If the accident is a minor one in an isolated area, open the window just enough to tell the other driver you would like him to follow you to the nearest service or police station. If he refuses, tell him to show you his driver's license, the car's registration, and the insurance information by holding the documents against your window, and that you will do the same.*

✔ *If he agrees to follow you, when you arrive at the destination, blow your horn for someone to come. Do not get out of the car.*

✔ *If the accident happens on a busy street, proceed cautiously, and try to enter a store or building or parking lot, where there are people around, to exchange information. Always get his license plate number immediately. If he is uncooperative, or takes off, use his plate number for identification purposes.*

✔ *Never open the window more than a crack to speak to someone. Do not pass any requested ID through this space; you may never get it back. Hold it against the glass to be read.*

If You Are Forced Off the Road

✔ *Stop your car, keep the engine running, and the car in gear.*

✔ *Leave at least a car's length between you and your assailant's car. If you cannot, try to stop where the area behind you is clear.*

✔ *When the assailant leaves his car to approach you:*

− *Drive away to a safe area.*

− *If you are unable to go forward, back up fast, and far enough so that he cannot catch you on foot before you start your escape.*

− *Pull out and knock him down with your car.*

If You Are Taken Captive in a Car and Forced to Drive It

✔*If you are made to drive the car, first buckle your seat belt. Assailants rarely buckle theirs in case they have to make fast moves.*

✔*Always keep in mind that you are in control of a heavy piece of machinery, capable of doing many things.*

✔*Your assailant does not know your intentions.*

✔*You have several options:*

– *Speed up to at least fifty miles per hour and jam the brakes on hard to throw your attacker against the dash or windshield.*

– *Drive into a store front (where there are no people to injure) and sound your horn.*

– *Cut off or even sideswipe a police car.*

Using your car just to attract attention is not enough. Your assailant must be in jeopardy of being captured. As in any hostage situation, your choice of strategies will depend upon how life-threatening the circumstances are. Whatever you choose, you must act swiftly and decisively.

Wise Precautions for Your Car

Of course, no one buys a car to serve as a Sherman tank. But stop a moment to consider. When you are in your car, as in your house, you do feel a certain degree of protection against accidents and against any aggressive, hostile person who might follow you or try to run you off the road. A car is also a means of escape or even a weapon against an attacker or a group of them. The larger, heavier, and more powerful it is, the better your chances for survival when you are in it. There are some foreign cars which are better built and safer than domestic ones.

✔*Cars equipped with automatic door locks allow you to lock your car as fast as possible after you get in. Cars with this feature usually also have automatic trunk openers which will afford you fast access if you need something in a hurry.*

Victims of violent crime, excluding the crime of rape, are more likely to be men than women.

> Vehicles that require warming up can delay your escape.

✔Built-in flashing distress signals will attract attention should you need help. An extra flashing signal which sits on the roof of the car and plugs into the lighter is even more effective. You can carry a folding sign saying, "HELP!—CALL POLICE" which can be opened to fit across the inside rear window. This is an excellent safety device in an emergency. With all the two-way communication systems in today's vehicles someone is likely to spot it and let the police know.

✔A burglar alarm system not only helps protect your car from theft, but some can also be activated by remote if you are attacked approaching, leaving, or inside your car, or if you are being followed.

✔An emergency CB (Citizen's Band radio) or mobile phone can put you in immediate contact with the police or other motorists.

✔A good CO_2 fire extinguisher can be very effective against an attacker if directed at his eyes.

✔Always carry two sets of spare car keys in separate places. They should not be kept with any other keys in case of theft. You can also hide a key in a magnetic key case (available in most auto or locksmith shops).

✔Keep your house keys, car keys, and identification in separate places on your person. If found together, they could lead a burglar to your house, and give him access.

✔Fully tinted windows all around will afford total privacy and prevent anyone from seeing the driver and knowing if you are alone.

✔A locking gas-tank cap will prevent your fuel from being siphoned out of the tank. Cars without this safeguard are usually the first selected by thieves.

✔A large, powerful flashlight, flares, and battery jumper cables should always be carried in your car.

Understanding Car Language

Did you know that your car speaks about you behind your back? Just as an attacker on the prowl tends to select victims for their body movements (see Chapter 3), your car is an extension of yourself, and projects much information about you. For this reason police officers often make sure their family car carries a sticker that identifies it as belonging to a law enforcement official. Having other law enforcement paraphernalia visible in your car can also act as a deterrent to thieves and assailants. Camouflaging your car is an excellent way to prevent crime against both yourself and your car.

If You Are Taken Away as a Captive

✔ *If it is at all avoidable, do not allow yourself to be taken to another place (hotel, motel, office, stairwell, basement, storeroom) or forced into a car or van. (See Chapter 12.) If this happens, try first to extricate yourself nonviolently. But this is highly unlikely to be possible, because this type of assault usually occurs very fast. If your attacker is intent on taking you somewhere, you can be sure he intends to rape and/or injure you. Once he has taken you, your options for escape and survival are drastically reduced. Even at gunpoint, the odds for your survival are greater if you try to prevent this in any way you can. If you are injured in the process, your life will still have been spared. And if you do sustain some injury, many rapists don't want someone who is wounded or physically damaged.*

When You Are Using Public Transportation

✔ *Be completely familiar with bus and train schedules to avoid having to wait unnecessarily.*

✔ *Make yourself familiar with all entrances and exits so you do not have to go looking for them should you need to make a fast escape.*

✔ *Have the correct fare ready so you don't have to spend time getting change, exposing bills, and possibly not concentrating fully on your surroundings.*

✔ *Choose the conveyance which travels the safest route.*

✔ *Never flash valuables, money, or jewelry.*

✔ *Distribute valuables in all your pockets. If there is a robbery, you may be able to surrender the valuables from only one pocket.*

Your car's physical appearance can be as "tell-tale" as your appearance.

In 1950 there were more than three police officers to respond to each violent crime; in 1990 the ratio was less than one police officer for every three violent crimes.

✔When you enter a bus, whether it is empty or not, sit as near the driver as possible, preferably within his view.

✔When you travel by train, avoid the cars at either end. On a train, the operator is in an enclosed area with no window in his door, which is closed at all times. He cannot see, hear, or know what is happening on the car. Try to find a car which is not empty, and with as many people as possible in it. Always sit near people. If this is not possible, try to find an aisle seat. Avoid sitting near a door or an open window. (Thieves often reach in to grab a purse and escape with it before victims are aware of what has happened.)

✔When departing, angle yourself, making note of the general environment, and the people present.

✔If you feel you have been followed onto a bus or a train, sit near or opposite the door. Do not get off at your usual stop. Pick a stop where there are crowds, or a store you can enter. When the door opens, wait to leave until it is starting to close. Then make a beeline through the door before your assailant knows what is happening.

✔If you are on a bus or train where trouble seems to be escalating, and you feel the driver (if on a bus) or others cannot help, get off and report the problem. Wait for another bus rather than ride it out.

✔If you are being followed off a bus or train, stop to talk with someone. Ask for directions. Then ask this person to walk away with you and explain what is happening. If you cannot find anyone, go to the nearest store, or stop a police car, cab, or motorist.

✔Keep your wits about you and look alert. If you are preoccupied, an experienced assailant can usually detect this.

When You Are Waiting for a Bus or Taxi

✔In a bus terminal be constantly vigilant, and avoid all isolated areas. If you have to use a locker, do so only when no one is close to you.

✔Stay in a well-lit, highly visible area, not in a doorway or near a curb. Angle yourself.

✔Avoid standing right in front of someone, but always mingle with others.

When You Are Waiting for a Subway

✔Wait near a ticket booth, someone in uniform, or the closest and busiest entrance.

✔Stay well back from the edge of the platform, and make sure you are not in front of anyone.

✔Do not stand alone; always mingle with other people.

✔Scan the area carefully. If there are few people on the platform, or if you feel danger lurking, wait outside the turnstile until it becomes more crowded, or your train approaches.

WHEN YOU ARE TRAVELING AWAY FROM HOME

Your guard is most apt to be down when you are away from home, whether on business or on vacation. Either you are preoccupied with important details related to your trip, or you are thoroughly wrapped up in enjoying yourself. This is why you should learn as much as possible about where you are going, how you are getting there, and the country, state, town, and area you will be in. Also learn about alternative routes. Become familiar with any important landmarks, facilities, or conveniences which you might need in an emergency. This holds true even for those areas you think you know well.

If you are going to a foreign country, be aware that assailants can spot North Americans by their appearance and behavior. Try to look like you belong. Dress accordingly, and do not act as if you are bewildered and in awe of everything you see. Of course you will want to take pictures or videos of the new surroundings, and to go shopping, but always use caution. If you rent a car, keep in mind that car camouflage also applies in situations like these.

Everything that you have read so far also applies to your new surroundings. But there are a few additions.

✔Try to find out about risky areas and stay away from them.

✔You will probably be carrying more money than you normally would, so take extra care in exposing it and securing it. Carry traveler's checks and use a money belt.

> *Alcohol and violent crime are not unrelated. Steer clear of people piling out of bars or reeking of alcohol.*

> Don't give anyone reason to break into your car. Stow all valuables, packages and clothing in the trunk.

✔You may also have more valuables with you than usual, both in your car and hotel room. Take extra precautions. Use all the safety measures that your hotel offers, and check them out thoroughly.

✔Prepare an extra set of ID cards, identical to those you carry in your wallet, and at least one twenty-dollar bill to keep in a plastic case. Store this in a safe place, so if you lose your wallet, or if it is stolen, you will not be at a total loss.

✔Carry your own portable travel door lock (available from locksmiths, luggage stores, mail order catalogs) and use it if you feel the lock on your hotel door is not adequate.

✔When you leave your hotel room, turn on a radio or TV to give the impression that the room is occupied, just as you would when leaving your own house or apartment. You might also hang the "DO NOT DISTURB" sign on the outside.

✔Do not get a street-level room or one adjoining a flat neighboring roof if you can help it.

✔Two dead giveaways that you are traveling are bringing a map into a public place to check your routes, and clothing hanging in the car along with other belongings. Keep as much as possible in the trunk.

✔When parking in a public place, position the car so that if you open the trunk, your luggage will not be visible to everyone.

✔Fill your gas tank at the start of each day. Do not wait for the gas gauge to drop to one-quarter full before looking for a gas station.

CHILDREN AND DEFENSIVE SURVIVAL PSYCHOLOGY

Many of the risk-reduction measures in this chapter also apply to children and teenagers. Parents can convey this information to them as soon as they are old enough to understand, but, of course, should do so in a manner which will not frighten them.

For children's safety, it is necessary to establish some additional emergency procedures. A first priority is to develop a secret language to use when each or both of you are in danger. Whatever words or sentences you choose to indicate action you want each to take, it must be totally learned. Each of you must be sure that when it is used, you do not question it, but accept that there is a real danger.

The next step is to establish ways that you would escape from an assailant, both inside and outside the house.

Rehearse your special or made-up words, together with your escape procedures until they are all down pat. Then routinely rehearse them so they will not be forgotten.

Just as these procedures can be used for the threat of physical attack, they can also be adapted to other dangers, for example in cases of child molestation, or fire.

Let your child choose "code" words. It will impart a sense of responsibility and control.

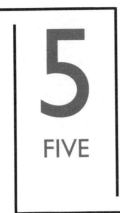

5

FIVE

Rape: A Woman's Worst Nightmare

THERE ARE MANY definitions of rape. The National Women's Study defines it conservatively, but consistently with the legal definition of forcible rape or criminal sexual assault. Rape is defined as an event that occurs without the woman's consent, involves the use of force or threat of force, and involves sexual penetration of the victim's vagina, mouth, or rectum.

SOME RAPE STATISTICS

A summary of cited estimates of acquaintance rape and child sexual molestation indicates that nearly half the women in the nation are sexually assaulted before the age of twenty-one.

While the overwhelming majority of rapists are male and their victims female, the problem of men as rape victims continues. In 1985 there were 123,000 male rapes over a ten-year period. In 1990, there were approximately 10,000 rapes of males aged twelve and over in the United States. It is still one of the most underreported and underestimated crimes in this country.

The paucity of information regarding this problem, the lack of research about the aftermath of male rape, and the absence of data for sexual crimes against men (until the literature began recognizing this crime in the mid-1980s) reflect society's image of the strong, macho male, secure in his ability to protect himself. Male sexual assault, therefore, is not readily addressed in our culture.

A 1992 government study reports the very scary information that rapes far exceed the numbers reported. The figure of 683,000 rapes in one year probably constitutes considerably less than half of all the rapes experienced by Americans of all ages and genders that year, since only adult American women were included in that figure. Research also indicates that the number of rapes reported to the police range anywhere from 10 to 20 percent. Other research indicates that only one in five to ten rapes is reported.

It has been estimated that, at some time in their lives, one out of every eight adult women, or at least 12.1 million American women have been victims of forcible rape, and 4.7 million women have experienced rape more than once. Rape is the most intrusive type of victimization, and the most physically and psychologically traumatizing.

I will not discuss the various state-by-state legal definitions of rape nor delve into psychological explanations for why men rape, nor will I offer the many conflicting classifications or profiles or types of rapists. If you are faced with a forcible sexual assault, none of this information can offer you anything to enable you to escape from your attacker. If you are being made to commit a sexual act against your will, that is what must be dealt with.

WHAT WE KNOW ABOUT RAPE RESISTANCE TACTICS

The various resistive tactics that have been advocated over the years have in many cases been successful—and will continue to be. In many others they have failed, and will continue to fail. All rapists are not motivated in the same way, and what may cause one to back off may incite more rage in another. In a rape situation you must evaluate your options differently than in any other kind of street crime.

All research suggests that it is difficult to draw any general conclusions about the best self-protective strategies in an attack. The situations and interpersonal dynamics involved are so varied, that to apply a single formula or profile to all cases would be simply absurd.

In addition, the research studies are inconclusive about the effectiveness of the methods used by survivors of attempted, thwarted, or completed rapes.

Among white victims of violent crime, females, and children or youths younger than eighteen, sexual assault was the most frequent crime.

According to 1990 statistics, American women were eight times more likely to be raped than European women.

People react differently when confronted by an attacker. We can do no more than speculate in saying that a victim's responses may be affected by such factors as her age, sex, race, occupation, social class, sociocultural background, marital status, and education; by such physical features as body type and build, constitution, and agility; and by such psychological factors as confidence and self-esteem, her attitude towards victimization, and her tendency to take or avoid risks, or be bold or timid. Her overall feelings of vulnerability or invulnerability will play a part, as will her relationship to the attacker, who may be a family member, an acquaintance, a close friend, or a stranger.

Other factors that will affect your response to an assault include:

✔ *The place of attack: indoors or outdoors, open or enclosed area (street, alley, car, house, elevator, hotel room, park, stairway, garage, roof).*

✔ *Time of attack: season, hour of the day or night.*

✔ *Kind of attack: whether you are completely surprised or are aware of something about to happen.*

✔ *Characteristics of the assailant: aside from what you can observe (gestures, behavior, attitude, speech, threats, intentions, violence), most of these are unknown. What you judge to be your risk of potential injury during the invitation stage, when the holding mechanism is operating, and during the confrontation and the altercation stages will all influence your behavior.*

✔ *The use of alcohol or drugs, whether by you or your attacker, or both, can all seriously affect behavior, judgment, reaction times, and general rational behavior, with resulting danger to you.*

✔ *The presence of others: pets belonging to you, people known or related to you. Every person will respond differently to the presence of others. Some may try to enlist their aid, some may encourage resistance, or some may influence others to react in a self-defeating way.*

There are conflicting views about how best to save oneself in an assault situation. Some advocate a nonaggressive, unconfrontational approach, giving examples of situations where a rapist was thus turned away from his intended victim, or tricked into not completing the sexual act. But this advice is not based on any systematic study of resistance, either verbal or physical, nor on any well-researched data on methods of deterrence.

COMMON RAPE RESISTANCE TACTICS

Some rapists have been known to break off an attack after being repelled by a woman's vile, sickening, or uncouth behavior. Women are advised to adopt a gamut of disgusting behaviors, such as urinating, drooling, throwing up, acting insane by sounding like a cow, quacking like a duck, eating grass, jumping around, singing out loud, or flapping their arms. But, if you choose to do something like this, be sure you can carry it off convincingly. If this is much too far from your personal style, do not attempt it.

Another approach that has been used with some success against rapists is to surprise them by being aggressively cooperative, taking the lead and initiating sexual overtures. This tactic has given victims added time until they could extricate themselves. In some cases it has terminated a rape, because the conditions were not fulfilling the particular rapist's psychological needs.

Feigning illness has also met with a share of success—but also failure. Collapsing and falling down, if it is convincing, or saying you have a heart condition, has been known to cause a rapist to back off. On the other hand, it could increase his anger, try his patience, and make him continue his assault more aggressively. Saying you have AIDS or a venereal disease is not a good idea. So many women have used this ruse that most rapists do not believe it, and some may even expect to hear it.

If you choose to mimic a physical disability, make sure you act it out correctly. For instance, don't grab the right side of your chest to feign a heart attack. If you intend to faint or collapse, as many women have successfully done, learn how to do it without hurting yourself. Practice slumping to the ground in a heap, slowly, from the knees downward, turning your body slightly as you do, and rolling over to protect yourself. Try to avoid landing directly on your knees or hip. Rolling your eyes as you go into your faint could also add to the realism. You might

Be smart and convincing when calling someone's bluff.

Rape is about aggression and power; a victim's fear fuels the rapist.

choose to moan or hyperventilate first a few moments. But once you hit the ground, don't move, no matter what. You want your attacker to think you are really sick, possibly dead. He might even think he killed you, and want to get away as quickly as possible. Stay put. Don't move a muscle, even if he tests you by poking or kicking you. By practicing this in the safety of your home, you will find the best method to follow, and get the "feel" of it in case you ever have to resort to this "last ditch" tactic.

Our most common reaction to an attack is fear, and showing it increases the likelihood that an attempted assault will be completed. The research that follows shows how responding with anger rather than fear may increase your chances for survival.

The results of research about rapists and their victims presents a very disturbing picture. I have summarized the most important findings.

RESEARCH FINDINGS ABOUT RAPISTS

✔ *Rape is a sexually aggressive physical assault against a victim, where aggression is the key element.*

✔ *Most rapists live in or near the neighborhoods of their victims, and may even be familiar to them.*

✔ *There is no way to distinguish a rapist by his appearance, manner, personality, expression, or by anything else.*

✔ *Rapists are deeply troubled people. Personality characteristics such as a need for dominance and aggression are part of their psychological motivation.*

✔ *Rapists use rape myths (such as all women subconsciously desire to be raped) to justify their aggressive assaults and avoid conforming to the law.*

✔ *The factors that predispose rapists' choices of victims are their own personal and social needs.*

✔*Rapists have psychological needs and traits that differ from nonrapists. They distort reality; their perceptions of a potential victim are biased to justify their aggression and their interpretation of the provocativeness, flirtatiousness, and attractiveness of their victim.*

RESEARCH FINDINGS ABOUT FEMALE RAPE VICTIMS

✔*Rape can happen to any woman, at any age, any time, and anywhere.*

✔*Those who are especially young, or are black, single, live alone, come home late, and those who use public transportation, have been found to be particularly at risk for rape by strangers.*

✔*More rape victims show submission rather than resistance, and repeat rape victims show strong dependency needs and naive trust.*

✔*The general public wrongly views rape victims as being particularly physically attractive, and to have attracted attention and assault by dressing provocatively.*

After surveying rape data, experts have given women advice ranging from suggesting they offer little or no resistance to urging that they resist their attackers with any means at their disposal. As you will see, the advice can be very confusing. Here is a summary:

MAJOR RESEARCH FINDINGS ON RAPE AVOIDANCE AND SURVIVAL

✔*Women can and do deter rape. They successfully resist violent rapists even in situations where resistance appears to be futile.*

✔*Despite the fact that women are vulnerable to attack, successful resistance can occur regardless of age, ethnicity, education, or lifestyle.*

✔*There is little relationship between the outcome of the assault and situational factors such as time, location, relationship of victim to attacker, and the woman's activity before the assault.*

The percentage of rapes has been consistently increasing over the last ten years.

> A passive reaction does not guarantee a victim will not be physically as well as sexually assaulted.

✔ Most types of resistance proved to be effective in some manner, for example, calling a neighbor, making noises, or engaging in revolting behavior.

✔ Statistics indicated that lack of resistance did not increase a woman's chances of avoiding rape.

✔ The least likelihood of attack or injury was where nonforcible resistance posed no threat to the assailant (reasoning, verbal threats, running, yelling for help). Forceful resistance using physical aggressiveness with or without a weapon was more likely to provoke attack or injury. But those who resisted were less likely to be raped.

✔ The more combined strategies involving strong physical aggression together with verbal resistance, such as screaming and yelling while struggling or fighting, were used, the better the likelihood of avoiding rape.

✔ Fleeing or trying to flee was the most effective but least frequently used strategy.

✔ The most frequently used strategy, talking, was ineffective. Pleading was ineffective as it acknowledges the rapist's power and domination, and the woman's submission, thereby increasing the determination to rape. Crying was also mostly unsuccessful.

✔ All women who did nothing to resist were raped.

✔ Women who acted immediately, aggressively, and vigorously were the most effective in resisting. Initially aggressive victims were found to be twice as successful in warding off a rape than those who were not.

✔ Some of those who described feeling enraged towards their attacker for even thinking of raping them were able to avoid a rape.

✔ No relationship was seen to exist between victims' resistance strategies and the amount of injury they sustained.

✔ No conclusion could be drawn that a rapist is violent because of the characteristics of his victim or her behavior.

✔ In spite of offering no resistance at all, some victims were kicked, slapped and punched, as well as raped.

6
SIX

The Trauma of Gang Rape

THE WIDELY PUBLICIZED case of a gang rape victim who became known as the "Central Park Jogger" has brought this problem close to everyone. Any woman who has ever been sexually assaulted by more than one attacker will tell you that there are no words to adequately describe the horrendous physical and psychological feelings that accompany such a trauma. This is because there is so much degradation, humiliation, aggression, and brutality involved. As such a situation unfolds, it escalates, with each member of the gang waiting to make his mark. Thus, a range of activities is likely to take place, including sadistic, perversive, and disgusting acts.

This is the most difficult of all sexual assault situations to escape from, because the psychology of mob violence is operating. Participants behave in this way because of two processes which are occurring at the same time. First, each mob member is subjected to more and more stimulation from other mob members, each being energized by the others and the victim. Each is egged on by various encouragements, and as the intensity and degree of stimulation increases, a more venturesome member will take the first step towards violence. The first assault stimulates the mob more intensely, until most members, even the most passive, have had their turn.

In addition, the action of the mob wipes out ordinary standards of acceptable behavior, and another set takes their place. These temporary standards have not been newly created, because the participants already

Only your wits can help you in a situation like gang rape. Physically defending yourself is virtually impossible.

condone this behavior. Any who do not wish to go along with certain actions are usually in the minority and afraid to exert direct opposition. Temporary standards of brutality thus prevail. This is exactly what happens in a gang rape situation, with one addition; a feeling of shared masculinity and power is also developed, exacerbating all the dynamics of other forms of male violence.

SELF-PROTECTIVE TACTICS AGAINST GANG RAPE

Although gang rape is less common than solo rape, the same precautions apply. But there is one exception in a gang rape situation: there can be no physical defense. The only things you have at your disposal are your self-confidence, alertness, ingenuity, cleverness, and ability to be convincing in whatever strategy you use.

Some women have escaped injury, even rape itself, by being able to identify and isolate the leader, and dealing with him alone. Many times a leader will readily identify himself in order to be the first to rape his victim. But if time has passed and he still has not made himself known, start focusing on the surroundings. Use your awareness and intuitive skills. Scan the gang and look for the most prominent male. His dominance, and how the others react to him will alert you.

If the gang is beginning to close in on you, you can gain time to get yourself together and formulate a strategy by asking who the leader is. This inquiry will usually be met with curiosity from everyone, including him. Once you have their attention, and he identifies himself, he will undoubtedly want to know why you asked the question. You can then go into your performance, and start playing up to him in any manner that you feel capable of handling. For instance, you might say that you prefer only to deal with the head honcho or top gun, or that you only like leaders, because they are the strongest, smartest, and best. Or you might try to convince him that you are so scared (this shouldn't be difficult) that you will be able to perform better publicly later on if you are alone with him first. Doing this will give him the distinct impression that you will cooperate as far as the other gang members are concerned, and it will play up to his macho ego. Even though he has the complete upper hand, he might still feel flattered that you want to be alone with him.

In a gang rape assault of three or more participants, there is usually one who clearly does not want this to happen, but goes along because he is powerless to stop it. This person is usually easy to distinguish and represents the group's weak link. Although difficult, another approach might be to play on the sympathy of this person to get him to intervene.

Your best chance of escape or survival is to convince the leader to take you away from the group, where you can hope to proceed as you would in any other sexual assault situation.

Gang rape can also occur when a woman is with another female. If this happens, a further complication is introduced, for neither of you knows how the other is going to respond; you both fear for your own safety as well as that of the other person; and you may be afraid your companion will do something to make the situation worse. Instead of being able to focus your attention on the horror at hand, concerns about the other woman interfere and complicate the survival process. If your female companion seems to have an idea, follow her lead, or watch how it is playing out. Stop if you see it is going nowhere, or if you have a better plan.

Do not try to pretend to be lesbians. This could backfire because the gang could demand that you both have sex in front of them.

If your companion is a man, different complications arise. Many gangs have been known to enjoy having the man watch his girlfriend/fiancée/wife being sexually brutalized. In this type of situation, either of the couple should try to escape. If the gang is directing their attention to the woman, her date should attempt to flee and get help. If the man is the sole object, then the woman should make the attempt. Nothing will be accomplished by choosing to stay with one's partner out of chivalry. Getting away as fast as possible to seek help makes the most sense.

PREVENTIVE STRATEGIES

Few women are prepared for rape and gang rape is probably furthest from most women's thoughts.

There's a weak link in every chain. Look for the one in the gang who seems reluctant.

Rapists don't necessarily choose the "best-shaped" figures; their choice of victim is more often based on personal preference and opportunity.

✔ *Consider discussing the subject with your boyfriend, girlfriend, fiancé, or husband.*

✔ *Go through your own scenarios for survival.*

✔ *Play it safe, and stay away from groups in deserted areas.*

✔ *Don't park in isolated places unless you can make a fast getaway.*

✔ *No matter where you are, always have an escape planned.*

7

SEVEN

Date or Acquaintance Rape

I DOUBT THERE IS a woman in existence who hasn't thought of being raped on a date. And with the escalating number of reported and unreported rapes women should give some thought to adopting precautionary measures in the company of men.

The macho male image, the need to "score" or "make out" has always been present to some degree. Society is conditioned to view sexual conquests of women as acceptable. In addition, themes of sex and violence are so prevalent in the entertainment business that the two are continually being juxtaposed.

DATE RAPE RESEARCH FINDINGS

A plague of sexual assaults has been sweeping the country. The most widely cited research on college campuses is Mary Koss's recent study, sponsored by Ms. magazine, of over 6,100 undergraduate women and men. It produced some frightening figures: 15.3 percent of the 3,187 female college students questioned had been raped; 11.8 percent were victims of attempted rape; 11.2 percent had experienced sexual coercion; and 14.5 percent had experienced unwanted sexual contact. Of these women, only 45.6 percent had never experienced sexual victimization.

Of 2,400 students recently surveyed at Stanford University, one-third of the women had suffered date rape. The coordinator of the Rape Prevention Education Program at the University of California's Berkeley Campus observed that female students have a one-in-four chance of being raped by someone they know.

The risk of a woman being raped by someone she knows has been calculated as four times greater than her risk of being raped by a stranger. (And nothing makes a woman more vulnerable to date or acquaintance rape than being under the influence of any amount of alcohol or drugs.)

AVOIDING DATE RAPE

Date rape is by far the easiest to avoid because you can usually see it coming—if you remain alert and aware. The majority of victims of acquaintance rape will tell you that the warning signs were there. All of them had a momentary suspicion, or feelings of reluctance and anxiety before the assault took place. Any such feelings should make red flags wave and alarms go off in your head.

✔ Before you get involved with any man, you should know as much as you possibly can about him, not just his "name, rank, and serial number." If you are meeting him through a friend, ask your friend to do some real checking—and don't be ashamed to ask. If you have met him on your own initiative, it is not hard to do some of your own checking. For instance, before making that first "date," casually ask him what he does for a living, where he works, and where he lives. Use this information to call his office on some pretense to see if he is really there, visit the neighborhood, and locate the house where he lives. If you are concerned about your date you can look into his background yourself. In the U.S. some police departments will run record checks or the information may be available at the local courthouse. In Canada, criminal records cannot be accessed by private citizens but be wary if your intuition is giving you warnings. The police may give you some additional safety tips. No one will fault you for being appropriately careful.

✔ Whenever you make a date, know exactly where you are going, in whose car, whether anyone else will be meeting you, and so on. If any surprises occur along the way, put your guard up immediately.

✔Be aware that the following events could spell trouble:

— Any sudden change of plans.

— If suddenly your male companion remembers he has "to stop off" for something he had forgotten to do.

— If you find yourself traveling on a deserted road, or heading towards an isolated, remote, or unfamiliar area.

— Receiving an invitation to stay overnight—anywhere—no matter how mixed the company.

— Being invited to his place, or being pressured to invite him into yours.

— If your date tries to convince you to drink alcohol or use drugs.

— If your date makes any kind of inappropriate or unwanted sexual advance, or overdoes any kind of physical behavior.

✔In all relationships of this kind, the cues you give each other are important. Whatever you communicate should be clear and precise. There should be no mixed signals, no room for misinterpretation. Your facial expressions, body language, the things you say, and the way you say them should all convey the same message. Teasing or flirting could be disastrous.

✔From the beginning, you must remain in control. If you choose not to use your own car, carry change for a telephone call and enough money for a taxi in case you need to make a fast getaway.

✔Act assertively, and set clear sexual limits. Your date must realize you will not let yourself be pushed around. Ask yourself how far you feel that you will safely be able to engage in sex play.

If you have been careful and taken the necessary precautions, you will be able to focus your attention on whatever message your date is sending you.

In summary, whenever you are alone with any man, until you feel total and absolute trust in him, you must always remain alert to possible danger signs. If a clear danger has been established, your decision to get

> Alcohol and drugs will muddy your perceptions and delay your reactions. Keep a clear head and stay focused.

out of the situation must be swift and irreversible. Do not be swayed by flattery, embarrassment, or a need for approval. Sometimes feelings of doubt get in the way of your ability to be assertive—guilt that you may have done something to bring on this situation, or fear that you might be overreacting—all of this must immediately be put aside.

Whether an assailant is a boyfriend, ex-boyfriend, fiancé, uncle, a friend's father, or even a stepfather or natural father, you are still dealing with rape and it must be treated as such in your mind and by your actions. An interesting phenomenon has been described in date rape situations: Many women who had a sexual encounter under duress do not think of themselves as having been raped. In the Ms. magazine-sponsored study, only 27 percent of the (legally defined) rape victims thought of themselves as such. But rape is rape, no matter what the circumstances.

> A person's level of education has no bearing on his propensity to rape.

RAPE ON CAMPUS

Everything about rape on the previous pages also applies to women on college campuses, only more so. Why? Because on campus women are always in situations that could be hazardous. Women's sexual well-being on campus is constantly put to the test, due to easy access to and frequent use of alcohol and drugs, "macho" guys looking for a conquest, frequent parties, the fun times and happy-go-lucky attitudes that often go along with college life, and walking around late at night unescorted. Also, the dorms are filled with careless students leaving doors unlocked, letting anyone in who asks without checking their ID, and so on.

In 1986, nineteen-year-old Jeanne Ann Clery was found dead in her dorm at Lehigh University. She had been brutally raped, sodomized, beaten, bitten, strangled with a metal coil, and mutilated with a broken bottle by a fellow student. The lapses in security at Lehigh provoked her parents to file a $25 million suit against the university for negligence. From that time on, the Clerys have launched a campaign against campus crime. They started Security on Campus, Inc., a nonprofit organization which has crusaded for college crime statistics to be made a matter of public record. In May 1988, their efforts were rewarded when Pennsylvania's governor signed the first bill of its kind, mandating that all state colleges and universities publish three-year campus-crime data. In addition, Pennsylvania schools must set clear policies about alcohol and drug usage on campus. This was the beginning, and has since led to passage of the federal Students' Right to Know and Campus Security Act of 1990. This act requires federally funded colleges to distribute to students, parents, and others their policies regarding:

✔Procedures and facilities for reporting criminal activities and other emergencies occurring on campus.

✔Security and access to campus facilities, including campus residences, and security information regarding maintenance of campus facilities.

✔Campus law enforcement: the relationship between security personnel and local police, and policies about reporting crimes to police agencies.

✔Possession, use, and sale of alcoholic beverages and illegal drugs, and enforcement of related federal and state laws.

Under the new guidelines statistical information for the latest three years about reported campus crimes of murder, rape, robbery, aggravated assault, burglary, and car theft must be distributed, along with the number of arrests for liquor-law violation, drug-abuse violation, and weapon possession on campus.

RAPE AND BABY-SITTING

One of the most common potentially dangerous situations for acquaintance rape is when a teenager or young adult is baby-sitting and, in fact, a large percentage of rapes do occur in this setting. Babysitters tend to feel relaxed and trusting of people who are there or come in, and whoever drives them to and from their home.

✔Before a minor is allowed to baby-sit a child, the sitter's parents should thoroughly investigate the child's family, and all the expected events and circumstances for that evening, including transportation arrangements.

✔The sitter should be instructed on the risk reduction measures in Chapter 5, and be checked on periodically by phone.

Verbal and physical assertiveness can be learned.

Children raised to respect their elders are more likely to be naively trusting of adults.

✔ Since most teens that I know tend to tie up phones chatting with friends, a rule should be established by parents of baby-sitters that at specific times while they are sitting, the phone lines must be free.

✔ An adult who baby-sits should take these same precautions.

8
EIGHT

The Self-Defense Rewards of Relaxation

WHY IS ACHIEVING a state of relaxation so important in helping us to survive a life-and-death trauma? The ability to relax yourself helps you to control your body, feelings, and thoughts. The art of learning to relax, therefore, is an important tool for transforming your state of stress to one of composure, so that you will not be powerless when confronted by an assailant. Relaxation will prepare you both physically and psychologically to correctly use guided imagery which will help prepare you for survival. Guided imagery takes you from simply feeling the confidence to control situations, to actually having the ability to control them.

Our minds are big bundles of electrical energy which can be recorded in the form of brain waves. These waves have patterns and measurable rhythms. During periods of sleep, the mind is in what has been termed the alpha state, working in a rhythm of about seven to fourteen cycles per second. We can also reach an alpha state while still remaining awake and alert.

Many people who have reported solutions to perplexing problems, achieved ideas for inventions, remembered things which they thought were forgotten, or brought certain bodily discomfort under control, did so in this alpha state. That relaxation works is a proven fact, and learning how to reach this state is your first priority.

We need to be relaxed prior to using guided imagery because relaxation enables our mind to be more receptive to the imagery process,

The key to achieving control over our body, thoughts and feelings is relaxation.

and to enhance its strength. The more relaxed we are, the more our sub-conscious mind can utilize the awesome power of imagery, and the more it will be persuaded that what it has experienced is real. Our sub-conscious mind does not question or analyze or judge the messages it receives; it just accepts. But it is very influential, and can easily direct the body to follow what the subconscious mind believes. Thus, when you imagine yourself performing an activity exactly as you would want to do it, you create neural patterns in your brain just as if your body had actually engaged in the activity.

When we are facing a dangerous, possibly life-threatening situation, our imagination works double-time, anticipating all kinds of horrors. This is destructive imagery. Such imaginings are quite normal, and you must learn how to counter them with constructive imagery.

You will find that learning constructive imagery will clear your mind, allowing it to be receptive to new ideas and all kinds of problem-solving possibilities. These positive effects will allow you to be more creative and enhance your intuition.

WHAT IT MEANS TO BE RELAXED

The idea of learning to relax, or of putting yourself into a relaxed state, may mean altogether different things to different people. To some it might mean sitting in a chair with their feet up watching TV; to someone else it might mean lying on a warm beach; to others it could be watching a horse-race, or sitting in a boat on a calm lake holding a fishing rod. But none of these activities can provide the kind of relaxation we are seeking.

First, you must have an attitude of open-mindedness and receptivity. This does not mean you have to accept everything you are reading unconditionally. It does mean that you have to be unbiased enough to adopt a "wait and see" attitude.

You must also be patient and give the process a chance. Most people today are used to immediate gratification: fast foods, microwave ovens, fax machines, and computers that give immediate answers. Learning to relax takes time.

The basis of all deep relaxation is paying attention to your breathing. This will have a calming effect on both your mind and body. Think of an instance where someone was in an upset, agitated, or panic state, and was told to take slow, deep breaths. Your manner of breathing sets the tone and mood of your mind and body. Many athletes (basketball star Bob Pettit and race-car driver Jackie Stewart, for example) use deep breathing exercises during times of stress. Meditation does not have to be done in seclusion. Some professional rodeo riders practice deep breathing before passing through the chutes on their bucking broncos. When you are upset, tense, or fearful, you automatically breathe differently than when you are calm, and so all relaxation techniques are based on using breathing in one manner or another.

BREATHING PRACTICE

You may never have sat alone and listened to yourself breathe. Try it now. Go to a quiet, undisturbed place, sit down in a comfortable chair, and just breathe naturally—in and out. Do not force it. Give yourself a few minutes. When you have finished, try to remember how you felt, if your mind wandered much, if you found it difficult. In these few minutes you have started on the road towards deep relaxation. It is as uncomplicated as this.

Now try it again, this time lying flat, placing the palm of your hand on your abdomen. It should rise with each inbreath and fall with each outbreath. Whether or not your abdomen rises will indicate whether you are a chest or an abdominal breather. The latter is necessary for correct relaxation. You can also tell which kind you are by standing (undressed) sideways in front of a full-length mirror. With your hands on your abdomen, note if your chest or your abdomen rises as you inhale.

Breathing from your abdomen is a slower, deeper, and more natural way of breathing, and ensures a smooth flow of energy to your vital organs and all parts of your body. This is how you breathe when you sleep, and how you should breathe whenever you do your relaxation exercises, or any time you want to calm yourself.

If you do not already breathe from your abdomen, it may take some practice to learn. Try relaxing the muscles of your stomach, or try doing it at first lying flat or in a reclining position, until you get the hang of it.

Breathing techniques lie at the core of disciplines such as yoga and Tai Chi.

Using a focus word
can help banish
distracting
thoughts.

You will find that, as you learn to pay close attention to your breathing, you will gain composure and a feeling of tranquility.

Relaxation provides another benefit: It allows our senses to function at their optimal capacity. Think how much more you are aware of when you physically and psychologically relax. Try to remember how much better you can smell, taste, see, and hear when you are calm, happy, and carefree. Then compare this with your senses when you are under stress, uptight, worried, and scared.

Relaxation is learned, like any other skill. It improves with practice and the more you use relaxation techniques, the more easily and quickly you will be able to compose yourself in an emergency. It's important, therefore, to practice relaxation once or twice each day.

You will find that learning this procedure is not as difficult as you might think. Since it is a natural response, it will be easier than many other things you have learned, and you will probably become confident of your relaxation abilities within a short period of time.

THE RELAXATION EXERCISE

The following relaxation exercise combines elements from Dr. Herbert Benson's *Relaxation Response,* a variation of Dr. Edmund Jacobson's method called Progressive Muscular Relaxation, and imagery. (See References.)

You will need a quiet place where there will be no interruptions. Disconnect your phone or use an answering machine. Lighting should be dimmed, and the surroundings as beneficial for relaxation as possible. It is also important to try to put aside your concerns so as to provide yourself with a quiet mental place.

Next, think of a word or phrase that makes you feel good, supported, or strengthened. It must be short enough so it can be mentally repeated each time you breathe out. This is your "focus word(s)." Here are some examples:

"The Lord is my shepherd"

"Shalom"

"Allah"

"Om'"

"Love"

"Hail Mary, full of grace"

If you choose something that is personally meaningful to you, this will be more calming than a less significant word. You will also be more likely to enjoy and practice this exercise regularly.

Everyone who does relaxation exercises will tell you that the mind wanders. Thoughts about your job, other people, your children, your parents, money matters, something you forgot to do, a trip you are anticipating, or a song you heard will come and go. Just accept these interruptions. Do not fret, or become obsessed with their interference, or let them upset you. As they come, let them go, and refocus your attention on your breathing. It is important not to put a value judgment on these thoughts, or think of them as "bad," or something that shouldn't be there. They are part of the process.

Interfering thoughts have been compared to birds which fly across the sky of one's mind, to be simply watched as they come into view and then disappear. Visualizing the words you are repeating can help you to refocus.

If you are in a situation where it is impossible to practice all the following steps (for instance, if you are with others), you might simply try to silently repeat your focus words, or visualize them in your mind's eye as you exhale.

When facing a traumatic situation, you will need the ability to gain composure quickly. You should, therefore, practice as often as you can in a variety of situations. In this way, your mind and body will become conditioned to reach a relaxation state easily and more effectively. It will be, in effect, like relaxing on cue.

How-to Steps for Relaxation

For best results I recommend listening to the following instructions on a prerecorded audiotape. (See Appendix III). If you choose to have them made, it is important that the recording person speak distinctly, softly, and slowly.

Begin by finding a quiet, undisturbed place. Get into a comfortable position, free of any tight or restrictive clothing. Let go of worries, tensions, or concerns which could distract you. Start to relax by closing

Don't be afraid to ask your partner or family for time to yourself in which to practice relaxation skills.

If you have trouble relaxing, try tensing your muscles first, then relax and feel the difference.

your eyes, and allowing your entire body to go limp. Now begin to relax more deeply by breathing slowly and naturally, without forcing a rhythm. On each outbreath start repeating silently the word or phrase you have chosen as your focus word. Each time you exhale and begin saying it, imagine a different part of your body becoming more and more limp . . . more and more relaxed. If you have not been able to decide on your focus word, as you exhale, visualize the muscles in that particular part of your body slackening up and becoming flaccid, like a tightly stretched rubber band suddenly loosening up. . . .

Breathe in naturally and, as you breathe out, silently begin repeating your focus word, or phrase, or brief prayer. And as you do, let your left foot relax. Picture in your mind's eye your foot's muscles going limp, the tendons easing, the skin becoming looser, and your toes beginning to droop. Again, as you exhale and say your focus word, or phrase, or prayer, imagine the same things happening in your right foot. Concentrate on the deepening relaxation in both feet as you exhale and repeat your words. Next, start imagining the tension leaving the muscles, tendons, tissues, and skin of your right calf. Now imagine the muscles of your left calf loosening as you continue to say your focus words and exhale. Imagine this relaxed feeling spreading down through your ankles and feet. As these relaxed sensations continue to deepen in your lower legs, imagine the large muscles, tendons, tissues, and skin in your left thigh becoming less tense. Now imagine the same for those in your right thigh. . . .

Start letting out the tension in all the muscles, tendons, tissues, and skin of your lower back and buttocks . . . in your pelvis . . . and around your genitals. Imagine the whole lower portion of your body becoming more and more relaxed. . . . Notice how your midback and abdomen feel as the stress and tightness give way to a loosening sensation in your whole abdominal cavity. . . .

Now shift your attention to the muscles, tendons, tissues, and skin in your chest. As you breathe out and silently say your words, picture the muscles in your shoulders and upper arms relaxing and going limp. Imagine the tension being released with each breath you exhale . . . in your arms and elbows . . . your forearms . . . your wrists. . . . Imagine tension being released in your hands and each finger, starting with your index fingers . . . your middle fingers . . . ring fingers . . . small fingers . . . and thumbs. . . .

Now release any stress in and around your neck . . . your scalp and forehead. Imagine the tension flowing out of your face, cheeks, and jaw . . . and out of the small muscles and tissues around your eyes. . . .

And finally, imagine this tension traveling from your forehead downward, through all the muscles, tendons, tissues, and skin of your body. . . . Imagine your entire body yielding to a feeling of pleasantness and comfort, as you descend into a deeper state of relaxation. . . .

As your body has relaxed . . . so too has your mind been soothed and become tranquil. . . . Indulge yourself in this mental calm . . . and derive pleasure from these feelings. . . .

Now it is time to bring yourself back to full wakefulness. . . . Mentally count upwards from one to five, knowing you will be fully awake and relaxed when you reach the number five. As you begin to count, visualize each number with each outbreath. . . . Now begin to exhale, visualizing the number one and becoming more aware of your surroundings. See the number two in your mind as you exhale, and start to feel more awake. See the number three, and become more alert to where you are. Picture the number four, and become still more awake. See the number five, open your eyes, and feel wide awake and relaxed.

Maximizing Your Relaxation Experience

Reviewing the results of your relaxation session after each practice session will help you to use them more beneficially. After you finish, try to compare the differences in your physical and mental feelings as you proceeded through each stage. If there were any particular times you felt better than others, try to ascertain why, and also try to find out what might have been interfering at other times. If you feel you need more waking-up time to be sufficiently clearheaded, go through the counting procedure from one to five again, doing something physical (such as pinching yourself) to reach full awakening.

APPLYING YOUR RELAXATION SKILLS

You need to get used to, and be able to transfer, your relaxation skills from the comfort and tranquility of your home to a variety of situations. You probably will not be able to go through your exercise uninterrupted, as you have been accustomed to in the solitude of your

Use a journal to record your thoughts and physical experiences during relaxation.

The more you vary your relaxation practice, the better able you will be to call on these skills in times of danger.

home. So, begin practicing as often as you can in a variety of settings, but do so only after you have become proficient, and feel comfortable and confident with the process.

Do not, of course, practice where you should be remaining alert and aware, such as when driving your car, waiting for a train or bus, or in places where danger could be lurking. Practice at work, when shopping, sitting in a waiting room, gardening, cleaning, cooking, waiting in line to pay in the supermarket, or having your hair done. It is very important to practice relaxation in situations where you are feeling stressed, worried, or afraid. You may even choose to vary the exercise at different times or in different situations, breaking it up into separate components, to suit your mood. If in some situations you are unable to use your focus word together with the imagery, it is perfectly fine to omit one or the other. You might even choose to omit progressively relaxing the parts of your body and concentrate only on using your focus word along with your breathing. Or you might find it easier to concentrate on your breathing and imagery without saying your focus word.

If you get into a habit of varying these procedures so you are completely familiar with them, you will not have to fumble around for the appropriate one when you need it. You will be able to either abbreviate it or shorten it on cue.

Migael Scherer was choked from behind and raped in a Seattle laundromat in 1988. Her book, *Still Loved by the Sun*, is a journal of the events of this ordeal. (See References.) During the attack, she was convinced she was going to die. She realized that she must relax and conserve energy to gain strength and time. In the grip of possible death, she knew enough to exhale and calm down. She willed herself to do this, and went limp. The detective on her case stated that in all probability, this is what saved her life. She wrote, "My life had pivoted on a desperate intuition that I should exhale and calm down. The advice I heard a hundred times in Alaska: In the grip of a bear attack, play dead."

Scherer chose to put herself into a state where a physical confrontation was virtually impossible. By doing this, she was able to provide herself with time to gain some composure. Throughout her book, she also refers to her use of special breathing in times of severe anxiety and stress.

9
NINE

Guided Imagery: Seeing is Believing

O NCE YOUR SKILLS and confidence in your ability to relax are fairly well established, you are ready for the next step: understanding what guided imagery can do for you.

Research has shown that through guided imagery you can change body functions which, in the past, were considered unchangeable through conscious means. Like relaxation, it is a technique that most people can easily learn.

WHAT IS GUIDED IMAGERY?

When you imagine, you are forming images of external objects which are not actually present. Although similar to daydreaming and fantasizing, there are distinct differences. We often use our imaginations for escape and wish fulfillment, controlled and directed only by whim and pleasure of the moment.

The "clinical" approach to fantasy creates imaginary scenarios that can be acted upon to overcome obstacles. That is what is meant by the terms "imaging" and "imagining" in these pages. If you were asked to visualize a specific object such as a door or window, chances are you could easily do so. This kind of visualizing is fairly mechanical. If I were to ask you to imagine yourself to be at a place and time in your life when you felt a certain way, to imagine who you were with, and why you were feeling this way, you would be using a variety of emotions, memories,

Visualizing your goal and acting it out in your mind is a sure step towards achieving it.

and thoughts, all relating to one another. I consider this kind of imaging "clinical."

For instance, if you are poor but imagine yourself in a dream house, this is fantasizing, an enjoyable kind of thinking. Similarly, if you have inherited a large sum of money and are planning the building of a home, imagining and anticipating everything about it, this also is imaging.

Guided imagery is a specific procedure with precise, clear goals. With it, our thoughts and imagination take on visual direction to enable us to feel better about, and deal more effectively with, past problems or painful events, and future hurdles and accomplishments.

Whether we realize it or not, we all use imagery all our lives without even trying. We use imagery as children before we can speak, and this happens as naturally and spontaneously as reaching for a nearby object. The infant who crawls around looking for his toy when mommy says, "Where's ducky?" is obviously retaining a mental picture of the duck in his mind. In the same way, telling a story or reading a book to a child also creates images in his mind.

When you explain to someone how to follow a certain recipe, or repair something, you are also imagining the steps to be taken. In order for you to describe what has to be done, you are mentally visualizing the process so as to be able to help the other person "see" how to do it. Think about a place that has been described to you where someone was on a trip, or did something interesting. As a result of how the event was characterized and portrayed to you, you can probably remember the images that were formed in your mind.

If those who grew up before television had not had the ability to visualize, they would have found that radio had little impact. Not only did the listener have to set the stage, they added all the props, adjusted the lighting, and dressed all the characters.

I also regard imagery as being crucial to understanding our feelings. It is easy for most people to form a mental picture of an event, complete with emotional associations and contents. "Seeing" yourself in this way allows you to look at your very private and personal attitudes, values, fears, thoughts, conflicts, and aspirations, relatively unhampered by the psychological defenses at work in your daily life. The expression "a picture is worth a thousand words," is true therapeutically as well as in everyday living. Using mental pictures is often the easiest and fastest way to find creative solutions to life's perplexing problems. It is language-free, crosses all cultural boundaries, and can be used anywhere, any time, by anyone.

Recent research indicates that guided imagery can help athletes overcome fears, increase confidence, and extend their limits. It has become the most extensively used training technique among this group. Not only the pros, but practically every Olympian athlete, practices some form of imagery. A few of the many noted athletes who have used it are tennis pro Gabriela Sabatini, a former winner of the U.S. Open; ski champion Billy Kidd; Lee Evans, the 400-meter Olympic champion; golf pro Jack Nicklaus; champion bronco and bull rider Larry Mahan; Mary Lou Retton, the first American woman to win an individual gymnastic gold medal; Greg Louganis, Olympic diving champion; Jerry Rice, star wide-receiver of the San Francisco 49ers; Elizabeth Manley, Olympic silver-medal figure skating winner; and Dave Stieb, pitcher for the Toronto Blue Jays.

Lee Pulos, a Canadian psychologist, uses imagery in his training of the Canadian national women's volleyball team.

The benefits of imagery have been extended to bodybuilding, and used by a variety of other famous people. Arnold Schwarzenegger, five-time winner of the Mr. Universe competition, used imagery from a very young age; Conrad Hilton had imagined himself owning a hotel long before he bought one; and Napoleon imagined himself being a soldier years before ever being in a battle.

Imagery is used in weight-control treatment programs, in the treatment of habit conditions such as smoking, and has been the basis of systems for improving memory.

> *Guided imagery can help you overcome negative belief systems.*

Overcoming Fear and Using Your Mind to Heal Yourself

Over the millennia, Native Americans were able to develop control over their minds and bodies, and, as the many stories of their privations indicate, were able to survive under the most trying of circumstances. Warriors, in the classical sense, developed a strong mind-set from their training in childhood and carried those lessons

Since ancient times, practitioners have believed in the ability of the mind to heal the body.

throughout their lifetimes. The first lesson the child was taught was how to control the power of his mind. By directing the awesome power of his mind he was able to overcome fear and pain. Fear, if not bridled, was seen to rule lives and had to be excised. Once a young warrior could control and remove his fear, he gained clarity of mind, and became prepared for any situation that would befall him. Fear could not exist in the mind of the true warrior.

In times of war, warriors would suffer great privations, pain, and wounds, all without the slightest complaint, even welcoming such discomforts with a resigned disregard. "It was the Spirits' will that I should suffer so," they would say.

To most humans, the greatest fear is that of death, the ultimate pain, and the imagined nothingness of the "Other Side."

Is there life after death? No one knows for sure. But ask those of us who have been clinically dead and we will explain—maybe. But, speaking of my own experience, death is nothing to fear.

From my extensive research on the Plains Indians, I have come to understand the power of the mind and how to use that power for my own advantage. I don't want to imply that I have been able to conquer all, but I have faced some frightening experiences and overcome them. I have helped to heal my body with the mental imagery I created in my mind by "seeing" the injured part, focusing upon it, and imagining how to fix it.

In 1963 I was involved in a terrible automobile accident. Both my knees were shattered. The morning when I awakened from my surgery, the orthopedic surgeon stood over me. With a worried look written across his face, he said "I am afraid you will not be able to walk for two years. There is a great deal of damage to your knees."

I remained silent for a few moments, digesting the terrible news, thinking what it all meant. Then I said, "No, I will be back to work in eight months." While I was sure of that fact, the doctors shook their heads and said, "Impossible! Don't get your hope up." But I believe nothing is impossible if one believes.

Two weeks later, I was released from the hospital. Casts of plaster ran from the tips of my toes to my groin, a most uncomfortable extension of one's body. (I was twenty-three at the time, and wanted to spend time with young ladies, not stuck flat on my back on a bed.) At home, I would ease my legs over the side of the bed, concentrating the power of my mind on them, and imagining I could see their internal parts. Every day I forced my mind to focus on the wounds, "saw" the damage from within, and ordered them to heal.

After six and one half months they removed the first cast. The physical therapist handed me a set of crutches and warned me to be careful that I did not fall. Another two weeks elapsed and the second cast was removed. Daily, I continued to focus my mind, ordering my knees to heal. Every day I watched my knees heal a little more. I was gaining the physical and emotional strength to be able to walk again.

I must explain that, soon after the injury, the State of New Jersey's physicians awarded me a 37½ percent disability status. This meant I had lost thirty-seven and a half percent of my normal function, and would be crippled for the rest of my life. But within two weeks of the removal of both casts, I walked into the doctor's office and handed him the crutches. The following week I was back to a full-time job.

The residual injury to the right knee was a net loss of mobility of five degrees, and to the left, three degrees. Although I cannot squat, having difficulty getting to my feet from that position, these are all the effects remaining from the accident. Both surgeons were so impressed that they used me as an example of positive thinking to help others in similar circumstances. But it had involved more than positive thinking, although I never explained this to them. I had used mind control over my own body. It was digging down deep within and controlling my brain to do what I wanted it to do to heal my damaged body.

—Micheal Joel Held

THE SELF-HELP USE OF IMAGERY

The power of imagery combined with a strong belief has not only been demonstrated in healing, but has been likened to miracles in other areas of living, as well. Whether you base an image on reality or not is unimportant, but that the image is strong and you believe in it is important, because a strong mental image can bring about actual behavioral changes similar to those you "see" in your mind's eye.

Guided imagery helps people foster feelings of hope and strength and overcome feelings of fear.

Avid readers of fiction may initially find guided imagery easier than others.

As was discussed earlier, our subconscious mind can exert tremendous force on us, both negative and positive. It can create physiological changes within the body, which can both heal and injure. It can also be called upon to help you out of a dilemma, or to make a decision, to achieve success, or to realize a dream. If you impress upon your subconscious mind the need to wake up at a specific time, you will do so. Your subconscious mind will often come forth in the morning with a solution to a problem which you requested it to solve the night before. We know that when imaging and faith have charged the subconscious mind with a request, circumstances have changed so that obstacles to success, happiness, or accomplishment have been removed. Financial failure can yield to financial success, and marital and interpersonal disharmony can yield to harmonious relationships. We know of scientists and inventors who have broken through mental blocks to reach solutions which came to them in a dream.

If imagery can help some combat their illnesses, it can help others find the courage to do what they must to survive a traumatic event. When feelings of panic, fear, and hopelessness arise, we cannot simply will them away, because the part of our nervous system that governs these responses is automatic and not under our conscious control. But by imagining things that make us feel safe, secure, tranquil, and untroubled, our mind and body will receive new messages, and react by calming down.

Relaxation and imagery techniques are not a cure-all. But added to your arsenal of defense tactics, they can be dependable tools. The object of the imagery process described here is to remove or reduce disabling feelings of desperation and paralysis that seize us when we face a life-and-death situation, and to produce and enhance positive feelings of hope and strength. In a critical situation, these techniques can help you to survive. Another benefit is clarity of judgment, which is an important element in making the right decisions.

Guided imagery can involve some or all of your senses, but it works best when as many senses as possible are used. To explore your capacity for imagery, a variety of exercises can be used, which consist of you imagining some different situations, and noting your reactions along the way.

The following "scripts" also work best if you listen to them on a pre-recorded tape. (See Appendix III for information on where to obtain tapes.) This allows you to keep your eyes closed, to relax, and let yourself become fully absorbed in this experience.

SENSING SCRIPT

Find a private, quiet place, and make yourself comfortable. Begin getting into a relaxed state. . . . Take a few deep breaths, and as you let each one out, let go of any tensions and discomfort you may have. . . . As you relax, let your eyes close, shutting out your surroundings. . . .

You are going to imagine several different things, and notice what happens to you along the way. . . . There is no right or wrong way to imagine these things. . . . There are no rules to follow. . . . These are totally your own experiences. . . . They are all about you, and can come only from you. . . .

In your mind's eye imagine a square. . . . Notice its size . . . how big or small it is. . . . Notice if it seems sharp or fuzzy . . . if it is constant, or comes and goes . . . if there are any changes as you watch it. . . . Notice if you would like to see it more clearly or vividly. . . . Imagine doing this with controls like those on your TV. . . . Play with the controls and see if the image clears. . . . Or just let it linger with you a while longer and see if it clears by itself. . . . Imagine it changing to the color blue, like the sky. . . . Now let it become three-dimensional, forming a cube. . . .

Let that image go and imagine a circle. . . . Let the circle change to the color red, like a setting sun. . . . Let it become three-dimensional, forming a sphere. . . . Let the sphere rotate slowly. . . . Now let it rise like a balloon. . . .

Let that image go and imagine the shape of a cone. . . . Imagine it rounded and solid. . . . Imagine colored stripes around it . . . red, white, and blue stripes. . . . Now imagine the cone spinning like a top. . . .

Let that image go and imagine you are holding a very tart lemon in your hand. . . . Imagine how it looks . . . its color . . . how it feels . . . its weight and texture . . . how it smells . . . its odor. . . . Toss it a few times from hand to hand, then up and down. . . . Listen to the sound it makes as it falls into the palms of your hands. . . . Imagine taking a knife and

Borrow an audio-book from the library and practice evoking physical sensations.

Your new survival attitude will positively affect your relationships with everyone with whom you associate.

cutting it in half. . . . Notice the pulp as it is being cut, and the color inside. . . . Imagine yourself holding one half up to your nose and smelling it. . . . Finally, imagine yourself taking a bite of it, and tasting how sour it is. . . . By now you are probably salivating as if this were actually happening. . . .

Let the lemon go, and imagine you are lying on a beautiful beach of pure white sand. . . . See the deep blue sky with puffs of white cotton-like clouds. . . . Feel the warm sun on your body, and the texture of the sand under you. . . . Let some sand run through your fingers, and from one hand to the other. . . . Wiggle your toes in the sand, and feel the grains between them. . . . Hear the roar of the ocean, the sounds of the waves breaking. . . . Listen to the noise of sea gulls above. . . . Smell the salt air. . . . You can almost taste it. . . .

Now release that image and imagine that your favorite food is being served to you. . . . As the dish is put before you, notice how it looks. . . . Smell the food, and taste it. . . . Hold it in your mouth a few seconds, and swallow. . . .

Let that image fade, and imagine that you are walking with someone in a garden surrounded by beautiful foliage and flowers of all kinds. . . . Smell the aroma. . . . Notice how you are feeling, and what you are thinking. . . .

Now let go of that image, and imagine yourself at a time in your life when you were feeling very happy, relaxed, and untroubled. . . . Remember where you were, and who you were with. . . . Hold on to these feelings and imagine them becoming part of you. . . . Allow them to grow stronger . . . to envelop you . . . to fill your mind and body with their tranquility. . . .

Now slowly begin to become aware of your present surroundings. . . . Let yourself come awake and alert, holding on to those untroubled and relaxed feelings. . . .

If you are making a tape, this script ends here.

Once you have become fully awake and alert, begin making notes of the images which were the easiest and hardest to form, the emotions you felt, the thoughts you had, any changes in mood, what physical sensations occurred, and if a feeling of tranquility emerged. If you wish, you may write these down in a journal. Referring back to it at different times will help you to remember and compare how your skills are developing.

The degree of change in sensation or emotion that you experienced reflects your capacity to use guided imagery. If you noticed very little change, do not be discouraged. Like the relaxation technique, this is a skill that can be acquired with time and practice. The more often you try to use imagery, the easier you will find it.

Remember, the more senses you involve the better, so do similar exercises to develop the imagery capacity with your other senses too. Try some of the following examples, or combine them to form your own special pictures.

In your mind try to hear these sounds: foghorn, barking dog, siren, crying baby, guitar playing, chirping birds, squeaking door, thunder, church bells, the roar of waves breaking on the surf.

In your mind try to smell these aromas: freshly cut grass, perfume, incense, wood burning in a fireplace, gasoline, leather, vinegar, chicken soup cooking, the ocean, coffee brewing.

In your mind try to feel the textures and temperatures of: sand on the beach, a metal railing, snow, fur, an ice cube, a football, a wood fence, grass, mud, glass.

In your mind try to imagine the *taste* of these foods: ice cream, candy, peppermint, a lemon, coffee, a banana, a grapefruit, sugar.

Try to picture yourself swimming, walking, dancing, running, biking, skating, playing ball, catching a fish, bowling, sledding.

Here is an example of similar exercises which combine a variety of senses. Imagine that you are vacationing in an old New England house in Maine overlooking the ocean. As you arise in the morning imagine hearing the sounds of a foghorn, sea gulls screeching overhead, and waves slamming against the huge rocks. Imagine smelling the salt air, and freshly mowed grass. As you ready yourself for breakfast, imagine the odor of freshly brewed coffee, toast, muffins, and bacon and eggs being cooked. You are also imagining how good all this will taste. After you imagine yourself eating breakfast, try to picture yourself in your mind's eye walking down to the rocky cliffs. Feel the wind blowing against your face, the irregular hardness of the rocks under your feet, and the texture of the cliffs as you touch them.

The mind is much more willing to re-live the pleasurable than the unpleasant.

Some people need an enveloping space as a place of safety, such as a cave, while others are more comfortable in the open spaces of meadows or mountain tops.

After you have done this, you are ready to learn to use imagery to enable you to survive situations where your life may be in danger. To accomplish this you must first get yourself into a mental and physical state where you feel safe, secure, and comfortable. Use the following script as you have the others (either read to you or taped), and practice in a quiet place without interruptions for about fifteen to twenty minutes.

The script that follows, called the Safety Script, is designed to decrease the state of fear, panic, and paralysis that usually accompanies a life-or-death situation. It is used to enable you to maintain your equilibrium and think straight.

SAFETY SCRIPT

Make yourself comfortable and begin getting into a relaxed state.... Breathe easily and naturally.... Take a few slow, natural breaths, and as you let each one out, let go of any tensions or discomfort you may be feeling.... As you relax, allow your eyes to close, shutting out the surroundings....

As you become more fully relaxed, imagine yourself at the entrance to a passageway ... any kind of a passageway.... It can be outdoors or inside ... opened or enclosed ... wide or narrow ... long or short ... angled or curved or straight ... level or inclined.... It can be familiar or unfamiliar to you.... Imagine yourself entering it.... There is some illumination from a bright white light at the end.... Imagine yourself walking towards it ... noting all the details ... the physical characteristics and lighting conditions, sensations of touch, and any sounds and smells within the passageway as you walk....

You are now about a quarter of the way through.... The light is becoming brighter ... and with the brightness comes a feeling of safety and comfort.... Halfway along now and it's getting brighter.... You are feeling good in mind and body.... Three-quarters of the way through now and the light is brighter still.... Feeling safer and safer ... more and more comfortable.... The end of the passageway is in sight.... As you imagine yourself arriving there, the light is all around you.... Brilliant, comforting, white light envelops your whole body like a bubble as it leads you to your special inner place of safety and comfort. . . .

This might be a place you have seen or been to before . . . in reality or in your dreams. . . . A place of total safety and comfort. . . . It could have been any time or anywhere . . . perhaps vacationing . . . or a place in a fairytale . . . or a movie, or a book . . . or just in your imagination. . . .

Whatever it is, accept it as yours . . . your very own personal sanctuary of safety and comfort. . . . Become familiar with it and with all of its characteristics. . . . Its appearance . . . sounds . . . odors . . . textures . . . shades and colors . . . temperature . . . how it feels to you . . . what feelings and memories you associate with it. . . .

When you want to return from your special place, imagine the passageway before you. . . . Imagine yourself walking back towards the entrance, bringing with you all those feelings of safety and comfort. . . . Now you're a quarter of the way . . . Starting to become more aware of your surroundings. . . . When you reach the entrance you will be wide awake, fully alert, and refreshed. . . . More than halfway through now . . . feeling more awake. . . . Three-quarters back . . . approaching the entrance . . . feeling so good. . . . Your eyes are beginning to open. . . . Going through the entrance now. . . . Open your eyes and come wide awake . . . to full alertness.

If you are making your own tape, this script ends here.

Take a few moments to evaluate your experience. Think of how you felt as you proceeded through the passageway, how it felt when you reached your special place, what thoughts and memories you were having. If you were unable to produce a place that pleased you right away, give it a little time. This is a new experience, and it takes some people a little longer than others to settle on one.

You might want to have more than one special place to use at different times, or change one for another. There are no rules, no right or wrong places. Whatever it turns out to be, it will be your refuge, a haven and safe sanctuary where you can feel comfortable and protected from harm.

Your attention so far has been directed towards using relaxation and imagery to feel calm, safe, and comfortable in a protective environment. Now you will learn how to use them in situations with acute stress or danger.

Relaxation skills can be used to lower blood pressure, slow breathing and heart rates and reduce muscle tension.

*You can empower
yourself by learning
to control the
outcome of your
dreams.*

Think of what you need to be able to do mentally and physically in order to survive a life-threatening situation. Ask yourself what kinds of inner problems or feelings you would need to overcome, and what changes would need to happen for you to feel in control should such a threatening event happen to you. With the use of the following script you can get yourself into a state of mind in which you feel confidence and courage, force and power, and control. Remember, what your mind feels and thinks will lead your body. And to keep your body safe is your goal.

The following Survival Script will help you to utilize what the Safety Script has prepared you for: using your abilities to escape.

SURVIVAL SCRIPT

Follow your relaxation exercise as before. . . . When fully relaxed, imagine yourself at the entrance to your imaginary passageway that leads to your special inner place, where you will feel more comfortable and safer in mind and body. . . .

Imagine yourself walking towards the brilliant, comforting, white light . . . Now you're a quarter of the way through . . . feeling safe and sound. . . . Approaching the halfway point. . . . It's getting lighter. . . . You're three-quarters along . . . looking forward with anticipation to that white bright light surrounding you, and the feelings of safety and comfort. . . . Through the end of the passageway now . . . Enveloped by that bubble of wonderful white bright light, as it leads you to your own special inner place of safety and comfort. . . .

Reacquaint yourself with this place if you imagined yourself here before. . . . Or familiarize yourself with it if it is newly imagined. . . . Take note of all its characteristics . . . its sounds . . . odors . . . textures . . . the shades and colors before you . . . the feelings and memories associated with them. . . . Be aware of your safety and comfort. . . .

While remaining safe and comfortable in this special place, you are going to let another image form . . . of another special inner place. . . . A second place in which you can feel confident and capable. . . . A place of security . . . yet of power . . . one in which you can feel in control. . . . A secure but powerful place of courage. . . . Try to imagine such a place as you did once before. . . . It may be familiar or strange . . . real or make-believe. . . . To do this you must imagine another passageway, similar to the first. . . .

Imagine the passageway before you. . . . It is like the first except for the light at the end which is a bright golden-yellow. . . . It is your source of survival energy. . . . Imagine yourself entering it. . . . The brilliant white light which you have already absorbed surrounds you like a bubble and lights your way. . . . You're feeling safe and comfortable. . . . Now nearly halfway through. . . . The golden-yellow light is getting brighter. . . . Feelings of force and power . . . confidence and courage . . . are emerging within you. . . . The golden-yellow light is strong . . . mixing with the bright white light. . . . Your feelings of force and power, confidence and courage are blending together. . . . Reaching the end of the passageway now. . . . The combined golden-yellow and white lights are intense. . . . You have arrived at your next special place . . . a place of force and power . . . confidence and courage. . . . As the image of this new place starts to unfold in your mind's eye, let the feelings of safety and comfort stay with you in your bubble of golden-yellow and white light. . . .

Let the image become clearer and more vivid. . . . Its clarity is unimportant . . . Your own special inner place to use to survive in the face of danger. . . . This place could be real . . . one you visited before. . . . Or it could be a place in a story, or from your dreams, or one you imagine anew. . . . Whatever it is, it will be your own place of security . . . force and power . . . confidence and courage . . . where you are in control. . . . Your fortress where you can summon your energy, muster your courage, and mobilize your survival skills. . . .

Stay with this image for a little while. . . . Become more familiar with all its characteristics . . . with all the physical and mental strength it is providing you . . . and what you feel it is capable of doing for you. . . . Begin to feel an added sense of safety and comfort from it. . . .

In this special place of safety and security . . . of power . . . and confidence . . . and courage . . . begin to imagine a symbol that represents this power, confidence, and courage for you. . . . Make this symbol your very own. . . . Whenever you imagine this symbol, a feeling of power, confidence, and courage will enter you . . . both your mind and

Having a survival attitude is a matter of choice, not predestination.

Being "good" in our society is often interpreted as being docile and submissive. Such attitudes run counter to a survival attitude.

body. . . . It could be familiar or unknown . . . human or nonhuman . . . mythological, legendary . . . a character in a movie, TV, book or play, a science-fiction or comic-book character . . . a supernatural figure, animal, inanimate object, or a combination of these. . . . Or you could imagine something of your own creation. . . . There is no right or wrong. . . . It is whatever feels right for you. . . . What emerges is yours . . . no matter what it is. . . . Accept it anyway, even if you do not understand it. . . .

Feel comfortable with your personal symbol of force and power, confidence and courage. . . . Imagine it working for you . . . becoming part of you . . . mentally and physically. . . . Notice where you feel it most strongly in your body . . . and where its power centers . . . in your head . . . in your chest . . . in your hands and feet. . . . Wherever you feel it the strongest is fine. . . . There is no right or wrong place. . . . Feel the warm, brilliant, golden-yellow light emanating from this spot. . . . Now feel it absorbed into every cell and tissue of your body. . . . Feel the warmth of the light getting stronger. . . . Imagine yourself amplifying it . . . turning it up as you would turn up the volume of your radio, and as you do, feel the light getting brighter and warmer . . . as the power, confidence, and courage become stronger, too. . . . Now imagine yourself concentrating this energy on your ability to survive. . . . Focus it. . . . See the light as it spreads through your spine . . . your nervous system . . . then slowly up to your brain. . . . Feel the warmth and power of the light as it travels through your body. . . . And as it does, feel your senses becoming alert and in control. . . . Feel your muscles warm and full of light . . . ready to respond with power, confidence, and courage. . . . Imagine this warmth . . . this bright golden-yellow light . . . empowering you to do whatever you need to do to survive. . . . as the light emanates bright and warm with confidence, courage, and control from your strong center of power. . . .

Now imagine yourself using this image in specific ways . . . ways which will make you more powerful and more in control. . . . Imagine yourself in different situations where you must use your sight, hearing, and smell, to detect possible danger signs . . . and situations where you must use only your intuition. . . . Imagine your reflexes. . . . Imagine an object being thrown at you . . . and yourself moving quickly to avoid it. . . . Now imagine another one coming at you faster . . . from a different direction. . . . Imagine yourself evading it. . . . Now imagine one object after another coming at you in quick succession . . . from different directions . . . and at different speeds. . . . Imagine yourself evading each one. . . .

Now imagine yourself using this image to feel forceful . . . powerful . . . confident. . . . To feel courage . . . and control when facing danger. . . . Imagine yourself in a dangerous situation . . . one you may have seen on TV, in a movie, or a real one that actually happened. . . . Imagine yourself facing an assailant . . . a mugger, or rapist. . . . See yourself in the middle of your bubble, surrounded by the golden-yellow and white light . . . the light of safety and courage, power and control. . . . Imagine your fear flowing out and away from you through the bubble . . . leaving your body . . . your head, torso, arms, hands, legs, and feet . . . and disappearing in the light. . . . Now imagine the fear replaced by feelings of safety and confidence, courage, power, and control. . . . Imagine yourself feeling them, feeling able to handle the danger. . . . And now imagine yourself actually knowing that you will survive this situation. . . . And finally imagine yourself using your personal image of force and power to overcome the danger in whatever way you can . . . by escaping . . . by talking . . . by fighting . . . by distracting. . . .

When you are ready to leave your inner places and to return, let go of this image by imagining yourself walking back through your passageways. . . . You have passed through the golden-yellow light of this last passageway . . . Heading towards your special sanctuary of safety and comfort . . . Feeling in control and confident . . . Approaching your inner place of safety . . . continuing on your way . . . Passing through the white bright light of your first passageway . . . Feeling safe, confident, and in control. . . . Approaching the halfway point and becoming more aware of your surroundings. . . . When you reach the entrance you will be wide awake. . . . Now nearly three-quarters back . . . feeling more alert and awake. . . . Approaching the entrance. . . . Your eyes are beginning to open. . . . Through the entrance now. . . . Open your eyes and come to full awakening, and full alertness.

If you are making a tape, this is where it should end.

Some people may initially be uncomfortable spending unaccustomed time on themselves.

SELF-TRAINING SCRIPTS

Honor your own power by looking for strength inside rather than outside.

Should you ever find yourself in danger, it will be necessary for you to connect with your survival abilities at a moment's notice. By practicing all the following exercises, you will train your mind and body to acquire the feelings of safety, comfort, force, power, confidence, courage, and control without having to go through the imaginary journey outlined above. They will appear automatically whenever they are needed.

First, imagine yourself going through the complete journey to your inner place of safety and comfort. Follow the Safety Script until it becomes routine and you are completely comfortable with it.

Second, imagine yourself continuing on to your inner place of power and courage. Follow the Survival Script, and do it until this too becomes routine.

Then begin practicing how to imagine yourself floating and flying to your special places, instead of walking. Do this by first imagining yourself floating through your imaginary passageways to your inner place of safety and comfort, and stopping there for a brief period to absorb the feelings. Then imagine yourself floating through the next passageway to your special place of force and power, confidence, courage, and control. Then return, by imagining yourself floating back from your two special places through your imaginary passageways.

Repeat this procedure but now imagine yourself floating through the passageways to your imaginary inner places without stopping. Then imagine yourself returning in the same way.

Next, imagine yourself floating faster and faster until you are, in fact, flying through your imaginary passageways and special places. At the same time feel all the comfort, safety, force, power, confidence, courage, and control that you felt when walking down the imaginary passageway.

Finally, imagine yourself repeatedly flying through the passageways and back again. Practice doing this over and over, feeling powerful, confident, and courageous as you do so.

When you have learned to do these things, it is time to prepare yourself to acquire these survival abilities instantaneously. Just as we can learn to automatically associate two words with each other in a learning process, the brain can also link signals with reactions. While still remaining relaxed, pick a secret word to say either silently or aloud to yourself, or a physical movement, which will become a trigger to activate these survival feelings within you. It must be something quick and inconspicuous: biting your lip, clenching your teeth, pressing two fingers together—anything that will not be perceived as an act of aggression by a would-be attacker. With practice, any time you use this movement you will automatically find yourself enveloped in your protective golden-yellow and white bubble. All your survival abilities will instantly take hold, your personal symbol (the imaginary symbol that gives you power, confidence, and courage) will immediately come to mind, and you will experience all the power, confidence, and courage you felt in the special places you created.

In practicing these scripts, imagine as many details as you can about your special places, using as many senses as you can. Commit all this information to memory or write it in your journal, so you can always bring your imagery back to it. Remember, whatever form your havens take, they will be your own sanctuaries from which you can summon your energy, muster your courage, and mobilize your survival skills. The more you practice this procedure, the better you will be able to experience the results, and these survival skills will be ready instantaneously whenever you need them.

USING GUIDED IMAGERY

Once you have learned to do this easily and comfortably, you are ready to create your own scenarios of assaults. In imagining them, do not limit yourself in how you use your creativity to survive. There are no rules on the street. Anything goes for your attacker, so anything should go for you when it comes to surviving a life-or-death situation.

First, imagine yourself flying through your passageways to your special inner places. As you are enveloped in the brilliant combination of white and golden-yellow light, imagine yourself feeling comfortable, safe, forceful, powerful, confident, full of courage, and in control. Now prepare to imagine your scenario. Just as you can practice your relaxation exercises away from home, you can do the same with all your im-

Treat yourself with love and respect and people will mirror these qualities back to you.

The mind and body in harmony are a powerful defensive weapon.

agery techniques. But you can practice these anywhere, even while driving your car, or waiting for a bus or train.

While still remaining alert and focused on your surroundings, imagine what you would do if all of a sudden you found yourself in danger. For instance, imagine you are walking in an isolated area, and go through a dress rehearsal in your mind of what you would do if you suddenly realized you were being followed, or if someone appeared out of nowhere. You can even imagine yourself speaking: how you would want to sound, the words you would use, your tone and inflection. Rehearsing routinely like this will help to ensure the future success of any actions you decide to take when your survival is at risk. It will also help to alleviate your anxiety and will condition your mind and body to be prepared.

Finally, imagine yourself at different stages of the scenario. It is useful to imagine that you have reached, or are reaching, your goal, and that your actions have successfully ended in your escape from danger. Suppose you have imagined your assailant in the process of attacking you. Allow an image to come to mind of yourself having eluded him, or of him in the clutches of the police, or of you being safe at home.

Becoming emotionally involved in your imagery on a multi-sensory level greatly enhances its effectiveness. Use as many senses as possible in your imagery (sight, sound, smell, touch) in all of your scenarios. When you imagine a situation, whether familiar or unfamiliar, imagine any odors connected with it, sounds you might hear, and the feel of anything you might be touching. Touch is very important to include since you are dealing with your physical survival. Imagine you feel yourself running, screaming, hitting, and evading.

You can relive certain of your imaginary scenarios and life experiences over and over, creating as many variations on a theme as you wish, doing things differently each time. By using the Safety Script and the Survival Script along with them, you will find yourself feeling safer, more courageous and in control each time.

Whether you redo some of the scenarios or create new ones, do not be discouraged if you do not feel right away as you hoped you would. It is best not to have any preconceived ideas about what to expect. Try practicing your imagery at different times of the day, and when you are in different moods, so that you may discover the conditions that are best for you.

Imagery Practice

When your mind is programmed to respond to a placebo it signals your body to behave as if it were receiving the real thing. Similarly, by practicing the Safety and Survival Scripts along with your spontaneous imagery exercises, your mind receives new signals which change your feelings, and in turn send new messages to your body, enabling it to organize and use its resources more effectively.

You will be surprised how fast your negative feelings become desensitized and dissolve into positive ones as the images are changed. Fortunately, it is easier to get used to the good things in life than the bad ones, and fortunately, this is how our minds work.

Imagery has the power to directly affect your feelings, mood, ideas, and thoughts. It can make you happy or sad, anxious or calm, fearful or confident, in turmoil or at peace.

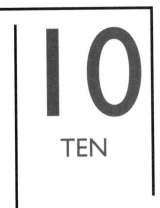

10

TEN

Disabling Your Assailant

Remember that it is always better to run to safety if possible. Physical self defense techniques are to be used only when you are left no other options to defend yourself. The use of any weapon, including the ones discussed in this chapter may be considered deadly force and can inflict serious bodily injury. You can be held liable for any damage you inflict on an assailant if the force that you use is considered unreasonable in the context of the situation you face. You, and you alone are responsible for the actions you choose in the face of violent assault. Neither the publisher nor the author take responsibility for the consequences of the reader's self-defense choices.

WHILE YOU HAVE learned how not to feel weak, your body is nevertheless weak and vulnerable in certain areas. But no matter what your age, sex, size, or strength, you can learn specific skills and techniques which will give you an advantage over your attacker. There are ways to incapacitate an attacker and keep him in a state of immobility long enough to extricate yourself, and make your escape.

You may ask, how can this be? The answer is by first becoming familiar with the most vulnerable body parts, and then by learning the proper techniques to use on each of them, from the various positions you may find yourself in. Because you might be positioned in such a way that you can only strike out at one part of your attacker's body, it is necessary to know as much as you can about as many vulnerable areas as possible. Figures 1 and 2 show the body's vulnerable areas. Starting at the top of Figure 1 and proceeding downwards, the disabling effects of different techniques applied to these vulnerable areas are explained in detail.

TECHNIQUES FOR DISABLING AN ATTACKER FROM THE FRONT

Hair. Grabbing the hair firmly, and pulling down at the same time, lowers the body to an easier striking angle. Enough constant pulling can bring the attacker to the ground.

Ears: Pulling on the outer portion of the ear, and folding it down can tear it from the body.

With fingers completely closed and slightly bent, clapping of *both* ears with the palms will create intense pressure inside the ear canal, causing damage to the eardrum and loss of balance.

Eyes: Striking the eyes by poking must be executed with a straight-on direct motion with the fingers or a small, sturdy object like a straight pin, key, or piece of jewelry. The eye itself must be penetrated for disabling damage to occur.

Nose: The nose can be struck straight-on, or upwards or downwards. It can be done with a closed fist, open palm, elbow, or a solid object. Any of these strikes can produce bleeding, blurred vision, slight loss of balance, and possible breakage of the bone.

Infra-Orbital Nerve: This small area located between the nose and upper lip is extremely sensitive to pressure exerted by a finger, hand, or object. Severe pressure can snap the head back and bring an assailant to the ground.

Mouth and Jaw Line: These areas can be struck with a closed fist, the heel of the palm, elbow, or a solid object. Hitting the jawbone from either side may break it, and will cause a sudden loss of body balance.

Hitting the mouth straight-on or indirectly from under the chin can damage the teeth, and cause a loss of balance.

Clavicle: A downward hammer-type strike to the clavicle with a closed fist (similar to the motion of someone holding a knife and coming downwards from above in a stabbing motion) will bring about some loss in the range of movement to the connecting limb, with probable breakage of the bone.

While the groin is extremely vulnerable, many assailants expect an attack there. Hair, ears, knees and shins may catch the assailant off guard.

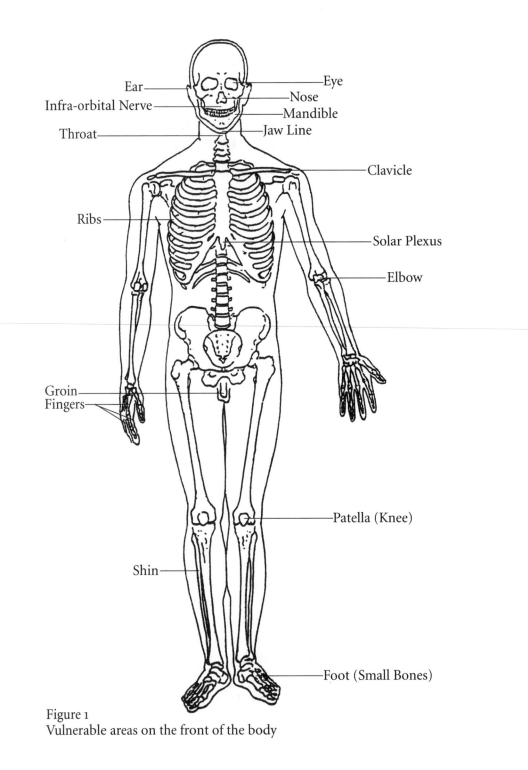

Ear

Infra-orbital Nerve

Throat

Ribs

Groin
Fingers

Shin

Eye

Nose

Mandible

Jaw Line

Clavicle

Solar Plexus

Elbow

Patella (Knee)

Foot (Small Bones)

Figure 1
Vulnerable areas on the front of the body

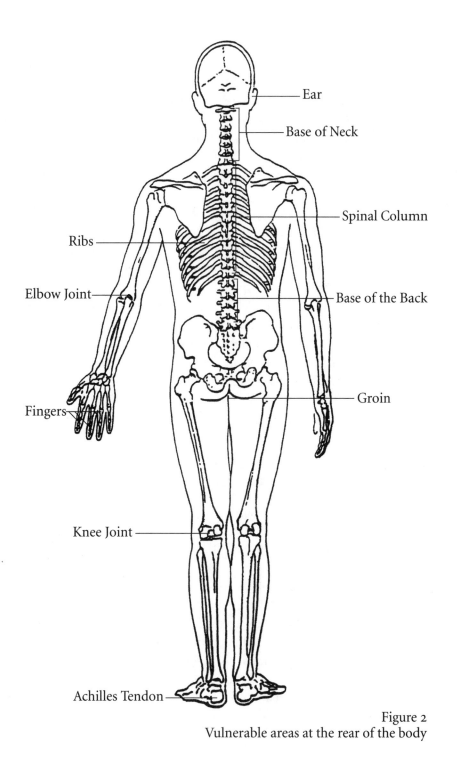

Ear

Base of Neck

Spinal Column

Ribs

Elbow Joint

Base of the Back

Groin

Fingers

Knee Joint

Achilles Tendon

Figure 2
Vulnerable areas at the rear of the body

Do not fight with your assailant a moment longer than necessary. As soon as you can flee to safety, do so.

Solar Plexus: Straight inward striking of this area with a closed fist, elbow, or bent knee causes immediate loss of breath, followed by slight dizziness, and a weakening of bodily strength.

Ribs: Direct striking with a closed fist or elbow can break ribs and cause a weakening of body stability.

Extended Arm: A hard strike with a solid object to the back of the elbow can break or dislocate it, resulting in immediate loss of the use of the limb.

Fingers: Bending and forcing fingers backwards against their joints may cause their breakage or dislocation.

Groin: Grabbing, pulling, squeezing, punching, kneeing, or kicking the groin causes loss of balance, movement, and stability, and bodily dysfunction.

Shin: A forceful kick or strike with a heavy object from the front or sides may break the bone.

Knees: Straight-on kicking or stomping of the knees will cause immediate pain, instability, breakage, or dislocation.

Feet: Direct stomping of a foot with the heel of the foot will break the small bones, immediately changing the attacker's bodily motion and stability. This works best with a shoe, but it also works with a bare heel.

TECHNIQUES FOR DISABLING AN ATTACKER FROM THE REAR

Hair: The same hair-pulling technique used from the front can be used from behind, but now the head is pulled backwards and down to the ground. Be sure to grab the hair from as close to the forehead as possible.

Ears: The same types of clasping and cupping can be done from the rear as from the front.

Base of the Neck: A strike to the base of the back of the neck should be done with a direct thrust of the elbow. This will result in temporary stunning of bodily functions, and loss of equilibrium.

Spinal Column: Direct striking with a fist anywhere along the spine must be hard and precise to bring about loss of breath or any degree of instability.

Groin: By angling the strike to the groin to penetrate from below and upwards into the body, the same pain and bodily dysfunction can result as when grabbed, pulled, or squeezed from the front.

Knee-Joint: A forward-thrusting inward and downward motion to the back of the knee done with any part of the foot can cause hyperextension to the knee and loss of balance.

Lower Leg Trigger Point: A straight-on kick to this point from the rear with the tip of any shoe will inflict an immediate muscle spasm which could result in loss of balance.

Achilles' Tendon: Driving the foot from the side into the Achilles' tendon and downwards with a stomping motion will alter the stability of the leg, in direct proportion to the degree of damage that has been inflicted.

THE USE OF COMMON OBJECTS FOR SELF-DEFENSE

Would you ever think of a glass ashtray, metal saucepan, telephone receiver, or pen as a weapon? Well, used correctly each of these could incapacitate an attacker long enough for you to escape.

There are several important things to consider, however, before using something which was not intended for self-defense. Any such object is only as effective as the manner and technique with which you use it. And any warning hint that you give your attacker will not only render this defense useless, but in all probability will produce more aggressive behavior from him.

The first thing to remember is to avoid letting your eyes rest upon the object in question until the moment you are ready to use it, and then you must not flail it around aimlessly. Your action must be swift and purposeful. This is where your imagery skills can help you immensely because they are the final and most important step before you act.

For example, consider that you have worked overtime, it is late at night, the building is almost empty and the office doors are all locked. As you are walking to the elevator, a man is following you rather closely. You are sure he is going to attack you. Ahead of you is a large pail of wa-

> *Be careful not to communicate your next movements through your eyes or body language. Anticipation by the assailant will weaken your defense.*

> *Do not be afraid to use as much force as you can muster; your assailant will have no such qualms.*

ter on rollers with a wet mop in it. It is leaning against a wall to be used by the night janitor. You decide that you will grab the mop as you pass, swing it at your would-be assailant's face, at the same time kicking the pail of water towards his feet. By imagining the method and technique step by step that you will follow, your body will actually mimic it as if it was already happening, as discussed in the chapter on imagery. The chapter on *Survival Techniques in Action* describes how this is accomplished.

The last requirement is that you make no attempt to use anything as a weapon—whether a baseball bat or bottle—unless you are absolutely positive you are emotionally ready and able to do so without the slightest hesitation. Even a split-second pause could produce deadly results for you.

After you are thoroughly familiar with the information in this chapter, start imagining yourself in the different situations depicted. Then go through your own scenarios for survival. You will be surprised at the things you never thought of, the feelings you never felt, and the ideas you never had until now.

With the variety of utensils, gadgets, and other objects found in the average house, most people will be able to find a number of things that can serve as defensive weapons.

The examples that follow provide a small but varied sampling of the kinds of objects I am talking about. If you ever have to use any of them, keep in mind that the shortest and quickest route between two points is a straight line. Always come at your assailant straight from the shoulder. Swinging your arm in a wide arc will reduce your speed, force, and aim, and will give the assailant ample time to block you. Remember that you should give no warning of any kind. Any hint that you are considering aggressive action could be fatal for you, so don't even stare at something you intend to use.

A large flashlight, folding umbrella, and a long metal shoehorn all have one thing in common: they can all be used either to jab or strike someone. If you are jabbing, the motion should be straight to the solar plexus, neck, or head region. If you are striking, it should be directed to the neck or head area.

Remember: Your intention is to give yourself time to get away.

Figure 1. *Hatpin*

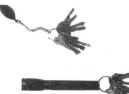

Figure 2. *Keys with object*

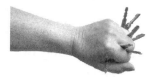

Figure 3. *Handful of keys*

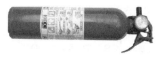

Figure 4. *Fire extinguisher*

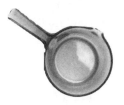

Figure 5. *Pyrex cookpot*

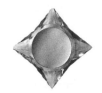

Figure 6. *Glass ashtray*

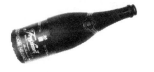

Figure 7. *Wine bottle*

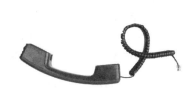

Figure 9. *Telephone handset*

Figure 8. *Candlestick*

Struggling uses up valuable energy. If one technique isn't working, abandon it immediately and try something else.

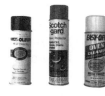

Figure 11. *Aerosol spray cans*

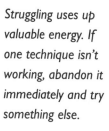

Figure 10. *Hair dryer*

The Old-Fashioned Hatpin

Figure 1 shows one of the most effective objects anyone can use for defensive purposes—the old-fashioned hatpin that great-grandmother used to hold her hat in place. It is long (sometimes more than six inches), sharp and sturdy, and can be concealed in a variety of places. You can stick it through coat sleeves and lapels, put it in objects you may be carrying, such as a book, magazine, newspaper, purse, briefcase, or shopping bag. (I know somebody who sticks one through the narrow end of his tie.) Try developing a technique that enables you to remove it easily and swiftly. Antique stores sell them, and flower stores or florists often use long pins for corsages. Even a shorter pin of only two inches can be effective.

It would be a good idea to have a second one as a backup. For instance, keeping a shorter one stuck through a collar or sleeve cuff would make it easy to use if you were grabbed around the neck from behind. Practice using them in different kinds of imaginary situations until you become proficient.

Keys

Figure 2 shows two sets of keys. One set has a heavy metal object hanging from the ring. This enables you to either hold on to the keys and use the metal object as a weapon, or to do the reverse. The keys alone can also be used as a weapon, by holding on to the chain and swinging them across the attacker's face. If you carry just a few keys, you can position them as in Figure 3.

Fire Extinguisher

In the home, one of the best defensive objects at hand is a portable fire extinguisher (Figure 4.) If you aim it directly at your attacker's head, it will definitely disable him long enough for you to extricate yourself from an assault situation.

Aerosol Sprays

Any aerosol spray containing fluorocarbons or caustic ingredients is very effective if directed towards an attacker's eyes. Once you start to use it, continue doing so long enough to disable him. One short burst may not be enough. Figure 11 shows a few of the effective types of sprays.

A Belt With a Big Buckle

Some years ago, a man's wide leather belt with a large, sharp, square brass buckle, called a Sam Brown belt, was worn by many street-gang members. When one of them was surprised by a rival gang member looking for a fight, he would whip it off, wrapping it around his hand tightly with the buckle exposed, to use like brass knuckles. Or instead of wrapping it tightly around his hand, he would leave a few feet hanging loose so the buckle could be swung. You can use any belt with a heavy buckle in the same way.

Jewelry

Sharp-edged pointed jewelry, brooches with straight pins, and heavy rings can all be used against an attacker to break his hold. If you are wearing sharp clip-on earrings, you might be able to pull one off and use it. Some women wear metal ornaments in their hair which may also be used in this manner.

Clothes Hangers

Even a wood or heavy plastic hanger can be used for defense if it is driven hard into a vulnerable area. The hanger should be held at one end, with the other end striking the body. When swinging the hanger, the direction of motion should always be away from the top curved piece with the hook.

Small Blunt Objects

Such things as candlesticks, a heavy flashlight, glass or ceramic pots, bottles, pitchers, ashtrays, a telephone receiver, metal dustpans, wooden dustbrushes, an iron, hair dryer, desk tape-dispensers, a clipboard, and a rolled-up magazine are examples of what can serve as weapons if used correctly. They should be directed towards the head and neck to achieve maximum disabling potential. Aim for the eyes, ears, or windpipe— your primary targets.

> *During an assault many victims experience feelings of nausea, irregular speech patterns and shaky hands.*

Larger Blunt Objects

Regular or folding umbrellas, baseball bats, canes, long flashlights, long shoehorns, mops, kitchen utensils, such as ladles, barbecue tools, rolling pins, and so on, are used in the same manner as smaller objects, but they afford you a longer reach. The primary target areas are the same, with all the rest of the body being secondary.

Small Pointed Objects

Scissors, nail files, the pointed end of a rat-tail comb, ballpoint pens, mechanical pencils, forks, knives, pointy tweezers, letter openers, and so on, should be directed at the main target areas.

With all of these your motion should be a straightforward thrust from your shoulder, not an arc with your arm.

Other objects, such as a beer-can opener, hair brushes, combs, and similar grooming devices, toothed salad tongs, and so on, have a more limited use, but can be effective if used correctly. Rake them over the eyes as forcefully as you can, if possible more than once.

There are many, many more possibilities. Check your closets and use your imagination.

PURCHASED SELF-DEFENSE DEVICES

Note: Before you decide to purchase any devices, you must find out if they are legal in your state or province. Before you decide to obtain them you should also learn when to use them, and how to use them effectively.

Mace

There are several different kinds of chemical weapons. Some contain the ingredient CS (orthochlorobenzalmalononitrile) and others CN (chloroacetaphenone). Both are effective. On contact, they cause a severe burning sensation and tearing in the eyes, making an assailant unable to see effectively.

Use mace only when you are sure you are in danger of being assaulted. If someone comes over to you, for whatever reason, do not suddenly whip it out and start spraying. On the other hand, do not wait to use it until you are caught in a strangle-hold. In most cases, you should be able to judge when the moment of danger presents itself. The time to act is when your would-be assailant makes the first questionable move.

Mace must always be ready for instantaneous use, and your use of it

> Being aware and observant can enable you to quickly identify objects that may be used as a defensive weapon.

must be automatic. This means you cannot keep it in your pocket or purse. No matter where it is concealed, you will not have time to produce it when you need it. Whenever you are in a potentially dangerous environment, it should be in your hand.

Mace comes in different kinds of canisters. On some, the front of the nozzle might be easier to locate by "feel" than others. If yours is shaped in such a way that you cannot easily feel the front, put some tape or glue there. This lets you focus on your escape plan without your attention becoming diverted.

But even after you know this, you might still use it ineffectively. In order not to accidentally get spray in your own face, but to reach his face, hold the canister away from your body, and point in the direction of your assailant's head. Most of these products atomize as soon as they hit the air, but some do not, and emit a single stream instead. It is important to find out which kind you are purchasing, so you will know where to aim, whether directly at the eyes and face, or in the general vicinity of the head. There are advantages and disadvantages to each kind. The single stream canister will be less affected by a breeze, and the user will be safer from the possible backlash of a spray. The atomizing type will have a broader range and be more effective if there are multiple assailants.

New on the scene of these propellants is one called pepper mace. It is referred to as OC (the food additive oleoresin capsicum).

Chemical maces are produced by a variety of companies, each with their own claims of effectiveness. Most important, the chemical make-up of the propellants and the other ingredients are not identical. This, combined with the varying physiologies and pain thresholds of different individuals, will produce a range of effects, some more severe and long-lasting than others.

Electronic Stun Guns

There is an electronic device called a stun gun, which comes in all sizes and delivers up to 200,000 volts of electricity. When its two small metal tips touch a person and the switch is depressed, the effects can be felt even through thick clothing. The shock produced is of such severity that it can immediately incapacitate an attacker.

When out in the open, be conscious of wind direction if you use mace or other propellants.

Before considering its purchase, you should find out its legality where you live, learn when it is appropriate to use it, and how to use it effectively.

Flare Guns

One of the most effective survival devices that I know is a flare gun—the kind that you find on most boats. It is legal—and can be used to summon help. A flare will always attract attention, regardless of the interpretation someone attributes to its use. It can be purchased in most marine stores and carried just about anywhere. They come in various sizes, some of which are so small that they can be easily concealed. It is an excellent item to keep in a car.

I strongly recommend that everyone, no matter how able-bodied, have something that they feel comfortable with on their person that can afford some means of protection in a life-or-death situation. For women, the elderly, and those with a physical limitation, this is an absolute must.

Be aware that legal considerations applying to the use of force for self-defense vary from place to place.

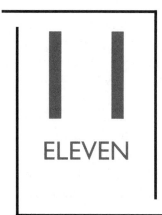

ELEVEN

Tips and Techniques for the Disabled and the Elderly

THE LATEST RESEARCH regarding victimization of older people indicates that they are less likely than others to become the victims of
virtually all types of crime. But those who did become victims were
more likely to suffer harmful consequences, sustaining grievous injuries
requiring medical care.

Some of the major findings are that elderly victims were more likely
than younger victims to face multiple attackers and those armed with
guns, and to report that their assailants were strangers. Those over the
age of sixty-five were the most likely to be assaulted at or near their
homes, and the least likely to use measures of self-protection. Among
the elderly, males, blacks, divorced or separated persons, urban resi-
dents, and renters were all in a higher risk category than others.

In general, elderly people's lower susceptibility to victimization is
due to their lifestyle of staying at home, the lack of a full-time job and
few regular after-dark activities.

Since statistics for crime against disabled people are not compiled
by any national government agency, the scope of the problem cannot be
accurately assessed. But regardless of the statistics, physically disabled
people are at a higher than normal risk because they are becoming more
mobile and increasing their exposure, while most are not increasing
their ability to protect themselves.

There is no way to know in advance how an attacker will treat a

Assailants least
expect resistance
from the elderly and
the disabled.

victim, or whether you will be more or less vulnerable to attack based upon your physical appearance. I know of a thirty-year-old, two-hundred-pound weight-lifter who was mugged and then pistol-whipped, and someone who walked with a limp who was mugged but not harmed.

Because an assailant is likely to assume that an older person or someone with a perceived physical disadvantage will feel more vulnerable, he will be less on guard than he would be attacking someone he feels could pose more of a threat. This gives the disabled or older person a built-in edge of psychological leverage where the assailant may make a mistake. This edge plays a most important role and, used correctly, could save your life.

Even if your response time or reflex behavior has slowed due to the natural aging process, there is an inability to use a limb, or there is muscular deterioration or sensory impairment, if you are able to function independently in society, then a variety of your survival abilities are intact, and a variety of strategies and options exist.

You can use psychological leverage to give you a distinct advantage. The best initial approach is to beg and plead not to be harmed, because you are not a well person, and are in pain because of an affliction, or whatever you feel comfortable saying. Take advantage of any disability, and play it up to the hilt. Remember, in a life-threatening situation, you must do anything and everything to survive, and ordinary rules of social behavior no longer apply.

You must lay the groundwork for a plan from the very beginning. Once your assailant believes he is more in control, and that you really do not pose much of a threat, your psychological leverage increases. You might even invent a nonvisible problem, such as with your hearing, vision, breathing, your heart, or arthritis. With an older person, these all become more believable. But whichever you choose, be sure you know enough about the symptoms so you do not over- or underplay them. Remember that using psychological leverage is a ploy whose effectiveness will depend on how convincing you can be. Do not let it detract from your inner attitude of strength, which is so necessary for survival.

A BLACK-BELT INSTRUCTOR'S ADVICE

Eighth-degree black belt Michael DePasquale, Jr., founder of the thirteen-year-old Federation of United Martial Artists, author of numerous books and manuals on martial arts and self-defense, and publisher of Karate International magazine, is one of the few experts who has devoted himself to this area, and teaches self-defense skills to the disabled. His students come to class on crutches and in wheelchairs, with disabilities ranging from blindness, cerebral palsy, and spina bifida, to polio, multiple sclerosis, and spinal cord injuries. Michael teaches that dwelling on your age or physical limitations only increases your anxiety, and detracts from and blocks effective survival strategy. He tells his disabled students:

Self-defense does not start with the physical. The key is to believe in yourself. This applies to every child, teenager, and adult with a disability. Never believe that you cannot do what others are doing. If you look at someone and say "I can't do this," you are giving yourself an out, an excuse to be less effective than someone else. It is important that you have a positive outlook and feel you can take care of yourself. You must have confidence in yourself, and that what you will do will be successful.

On the physical side there are things that a disabled person can do, even that a disabled child can do. When someone grabs you, it is important you understand his vulnerable targets: throat, eyes, groin, kneecaps, shins. It is important for someone who is disabled and frightened to use whatever physical ability they have, and understand, for example, "OK, I can't use one arm, but I can use the other. I am not totally able to protect myself, but I am physically able with one arm to do something."

It is common for disabled people to have a negative attitude about their ability to defend themselves. Many people feel this way because they have never had anyone tell them or show them they are capable. I remember giving a demonstration where there was a sixteen-year-old girl who had been born without legs. She

You do not have to be a martial arts expert to be able to defend yourself from physical attack.

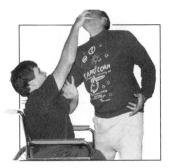

didn't even want to watch what was going on. I went over to her afterwards and asked why she didn't want to face us. She said, "Because I can't do that, and I never will be able to do that, and I don't like to look at things I really believe I can't do. It depresses me." So I said to her, "What makes you think you can't do this?" She said, "Because I have no legs." So I said, "Well, you have arms."

I took her aside and said, "Let me show you something, and never forget this as long as you live. If someone attacks you, for the most part they will always come in close to you. You have the ability to grab, to strike. Do you know you have the ability to do that? Do you have the ability to pick up a fork, a pen? Do you have the ability to iron your clothes, to fold your clothes? Sure you have no legs, but do you have these abilities?" She said, "Yes." "Then you have the ability to do anything, maybe not as well as some people, but you can learn."

Then I had a few students come over and grab her by the throat, by the wrists, and I showed her a few different techniques, very workable techniques for her. She was amazed.

I've walked into a class of thirty-five disabled people who were there just out of curiosity, and they were all there with a negative attitude. At first, a good 25 percent of them would just sit and do nothing. Eventually most of them saw how this can work, and started to believe in themselves.

As a disabled person, you want to be able to go anywhere like everybody else, and not feel you're an easy prey. You want to be as confident and secure as possible when you get on the street, whether you are in a wheelchair or not. The people who help you learn to defend yourself can only inspire you to the degree that you let yourself be inspired. While ability is in all of us, energy, desire, and enthusiasm are not.

The inspiration or desire to help yourself will not come from lectures, pep talks, or even from this book. But the fact that you are taking the time to read this indicates that you feel it is important to you. Please understand that you do not have to be an easy prey, and that disability is not synonymous with victimization. Now, ask yourself, "Is it important enough for me to allocate the time to take care of myself, because of the situation I'm in? Is it time to do something about my vulnerability?" If the answer is "yes," then you will have to make time available.

There are progressive stages to self-defense. First, you have to understand your environment and how to protect yourself with environmental awareness.

When an assailant attacks, he is looking for a victim, not an opponent. The next step is understanding how a disabled person is seen as an easier prey than others, and how effective the elements of surprise and resistance can be coming from such a person.

An essential part of Michael's program emphasizes the importance of family members' and friends' support and encouragement:

> Knowing others are behind you saying "You can do it," is what is necessary if the inspiration, enthusiasm, energy, and desire are to be nurtured. Search out situations where they exist. Those who surround disabled people, spending time and working with them, can provide the encouragement they need to follow through on practicing, physically and mentally, how to secure themselves out there. This has been instrumental in our success.

DEFENSE TACTICS IF YOU ARE ON CRUTCHES OR IN A WHEELCHAIR

Michael advocates that all disabled people carry some protective device on their persons. Whatever you choose, you should become thoroughly familiar with its usage. I recommend you carry more than one, so you have a back-up in case one is taken away. It could be a rattail comb, keys on a long chain, a hat pin, or a screwdriver. It could be mace, a stick or club, or a pointed object. Any object that resembles a weapon should be kept hidden until its moment of use.

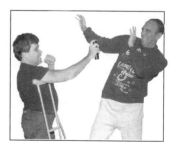

If you are in a wheelchair, keep such objects close to your outer thigh, easily accessible to your hand. Objects such as a folding umbrella, a rolled-up magazine, or keys can be kept where they are visible.

If someone aggressive approaches you, put your hands down at your side while you negotiate and try to avoid a physical confrontation, but

The only real limitations in life are the ones in your mind.

at the same time grasp your weapon. Do not expose it until the assailant has become committed to attack and actually comes at you. Though it can be easier to take a weapon away from someone who is disabled, because their center of balance is less secure, this does not justify not using one. But it is why it is crucial that a weapon be exposed and used at the last possible moment. At the moment the assailant is coming at you, the stick can come up to whack him across the head, or jab him in the groin, or in the neck.

Practice how to respond to an attacker by sitting in front of a mirror with the weapon in your hand. A stick or club can be held in two ways: First, with three-quarters of it protruding from the hand, your swing starts from the shoulder proceeding in an arc as if you were using a whip. You bring it all the way back, and then the shoulder, the elbow, and the wrist all swing the stick forward. The second way to hold the stick is with only about three inches protruding from the hand, and the rest of it underneath and against the blade of the arm. This way you can still jab forward, and also defend yourself from a knife or club attack by blocking it with the protected side of your arm. After you block the weapon, you can flick the stick out and forward into your assailant's neck, face, or head, and extend the stick from your hand to hit him across the face or head. Use your imagery skills to visualize these moves in various situations and environments.

Almost inevitably someone in a wheelchair or on crutches will wind up on the ground. So it is important to practice how to fall without getting hurt by using your hands and the fleshy part of the forearm to slap the ground as you fall, holding your face back. You should also learn how to use the ground to your advantage. Practice defending yourself from this position by using the stick like a dagger, as if jamming it into the foot, slapping the knees, and jabbing into the groin if you can reach that high. If your attacker goes down, use it to strike the head or neck.

If you are using crutches or a cane, you have an advantage over someone in a wheelchair only because you are already holding on to a stick and it is a longer stick. The disadvantage is that it is harder to control, but it is used in the same way. Again, practice your moves in front of a mirror, and by using imagery. Practice striking to the knees, thrusting to the solar plexus, the throat, eyes, and temples. It is important to learn to use whipping, hooking, and back-slashing motions, because you never know when one of these might be necessary.

If you have a heavy bag, you can use it as a target to practice your swings and punches using your body parts, as well as smacking it with the cane or crutch. Since constant hitting will probably break or weaken your cane or crutch, it is advisable to practice with an old crutch, broom handle, or a heavy club.

You can also put tape on various areas of the bag to help target your strikes. Tape Xs on the bag for the assailant's eyes, throat, groin, and other vulnerable body parts. If you are creative, you might want to paint parts of the body on the bag to help increase your precision, and add some realism to the whole process. Practice hooking, back-slashing, swinging up, coming down over the head, and thrusting straight into it. You can also practice hitting the bag from the ground. The purpose of these exercises is to get you used to focusing on and knowing how it feels to hit something.

A weapon can give you some distance, so your assailant cannot get close to you, but remember that if you lose your cane, crutch, or stick, they are actually extensions of your arm and hand, and that anything you can do with them you can also do with your hand. If an attacker (without a gun) is out to harm you, he is going to have to get close enough to do so, and once he is close enough, if you are secure, focused, and skilled in self-defense techniques, even if you are disabled you can have a significant advantage over him.

When you first start to practice some of these techniques, you will probably be a little sore. After all, you will be using muscles you haven't used for a long time. This is good for you both physically and psychologically. Though people on crutches or in a wheelchair cannot use the energy in their legs and hips for leverage, they can compensate by making their upper bodies incredibly strong. You can accomplish this by doing dips in the wheelchair, crawling across a room using your forearms and elbows, or any parts of the body you can use, doing curls (lifting weights with the forearm), and any other exercises you are comfortable with. This will help strengthen various areas of your body, and enable them to move with force if they have to.

Surround yourself with positive thinkers; negative people will only drag you down.

Hearing and smell are powerful senses that visually impaired people can rely on to augment their defense.

Use your imagery skills while doing everything that has been described.

DEFENSE TACTICS IF YOU ARE VISUALLY IMPAIRED

If you are visually impaired, there are other techniques that you can learn. Finding someone to train with will be essential, beginning with their reading this book to you. For those interested in self-defense training, I would suggest you start by contacting some local martial arts schools. If no programs are available there, contact state or national organizations. More martial arts programs for those with special needs are coming into existence. You might even seek out a qualified instructor who is willing to start a group program for you and others.

The most important thing for you to learn is how to feel another's body, and know with only a second's touch exactly what part of the body you are touching. You should learn to be able to tell how far away from you the other person is. Are his knees within reach of your cane? Is he coming closer or moving away? A good exercise that develops this skill is for you to stand still, while the other person talks, moves, and makes noises at varying distances and volumes.

Another exercise is to have a mock assailant try an attack. In this way, you can become accustomed to finding certain vulnerable areas of the assailant's body and to practice certain moves. You can practice blocking the assailant, feeling him, sliding up your arm to reach his throat and head region. Once you locate an arm, you will know where every other part of the body is.

Keep in mind that most visually impaired people (depending upon age at the onset) can use imagery skills as effectively as anyone with normal vision. Imagining is in the mind, not in the eye—remember the expression "seeing with your mind's eye?" For many visually impaired people, imagery can be a very strong, useful, and effective aid.

In the event that you lose your glasses during an assault, try practicing without them the exercises recommended for those with more limited vision.

PROFESSIONAL SELF-DEFENSE TRAINING

The choice of whether to pursue defensive training is a very personal and individual one. But many disabled people who have decided to take this route have reported remarkable results, both physically and psychologically. Two of Michael's students have consented to write about their experiences in the hope that their message will help other disabled people.

The first commentary is by Richard Diamond, a professional social worker in his thirties, who works with physically handicapped children and their families. He was born with spina bifida and must walk with crutches. As of this writing, Richard has received his black belt in ju-jitsu.

RICHARD'S SELF-DEFENSE TIPS

In my own as well as other disabled people's minds exist two fundamental questions: "If I'm attacked, can I defend myself?" and "Will I defend myself?" There are only two options: to submit or to defend yourself. Each of these two options, if used correctly, can be effective in saving your life. In my own lifetime, I have experienced confrontations that have resulted in physical altercations. I have also been able to prevent such encounters. Whether being confronted or attacked, I have always emerged unscathed, with my dignity and body intact, because of the techniques I have learned to use in everyday living. These techniques can be used by anyone, regardless of disability. All you have to do to make them work for you is to have a desire to defend yourself, and the belief that you are someone who deserves to be treated with respect and dignity.

Listing Your Fears

Make a list of your fears; let's say you fear being attacked. Now take this word and break it down into categories of what it means to you and how it makes you afraid. At this point it is just a word, a very stressful one. Just for example, let's say the words you associate with the word

Listing your fears and analyzing them one by one can help you focus on how to reduce your risks.

Your activities need not be limited by your fears, as long as you take the time to make plans for your safety beforehand.

"attack" are pain, helplessness, anger, insecurity, violation, and abuse. I want you to know that these fears exist in all people, not only in those who are disabled.

After you have made your own list of associated words, focus first on the least stressful one. Using my list, I'll pick insecurity, the feeling of being insecure, which I will define for myself as feeling robbed. I think of those objects I normally carry and think how it would feel if any of them were to be taken away. When you try this, think how would this affect your life? Can any of them be replaced? Once you realize how seriously concerned you are about losing an irreplaceable possession, you will not carry it with you in dangerous areas. This kind of thinking can help you to worry less and relax more.

Now continue on to the other words I have listed. They all are related to your emotions. In order for you to be able to face an attacker in the real world without being overwhelmed by your fears, you have to look inside and explore your inner self.

Listing Your Best Qualities

Continue your list, writing down everything you feel is positive about yourself. Then ask some friends to tell you what they see as your positive attributes. Go over this list a few times each day until you believe, just as others do, that you have good qualities, and that these are among the reasons for you to protect yourself from attack.

Listing Your Daily Activities

The next step is to simply admit that you don't like pain, and that you are afraid of being attacked, just like everyone else. This leads to the list of all your daily activities: where you go and what you do each day. Write "Home safe" at the end of each day's list.

Review this list at the beginning and end of each day. This will help you to see that you can go out in the world and arrive at your destination safely without always fearing you will be attacked. Most disabled people are fearful of going outside alone and not getting home safely. It is a fear which has developed not just from their own or others' experience, but rather from what they have seen on TV or read about. By writing this list, you can deal with these fears on a different level. Writing them enables you to look at them from a different perspective, especially when you arrive home unharmed, and see that they are unreal. This procedure can also prepare you to deal with your safety concerns about going to other places.

You cannot totally prevent yourself from being attacked, but you can minimize the chances of it happening. Facing your fears will prevent you from becoming a prisoner in your mind.

Planning Your Day

The first steps in preparing yourself for any kind of confrontation are to develop mental concentration and an effective ongoing routine. This means that you should develop specific tasks to be done on a daily basis, beginning from the time of arising in the morning, and continuing through the planning of the day's activities. For instance, whom you will contact before leaving the house, what you will do before leaving, such as writing down directions, getting phone numbers of places you will be going, mapping out directions, checking on road, weather, and car conditions. How long it will take you to develop this routine can vary according to your present mental state, your past experiences in the outside world, your home environment, and your degree of determination. Regardless of the past, you can take control of the present and future without any outside help. I will assume that if you have read this far, you do have the determination!

Once you are less burdened by fear, the next step is to minimize your chances of being confronted or assaulted. You can accomplish this by first planning your day. Include everything you will be doing and where you will be going, with the routes you will be traveling and the time it should take you. Whether you must go through a familiar area, or one you know is unsafe, or are headed for a place you have never been before, the preparations will be the same:

If you are using your own transportation, make sure your car is in good working condition. Carry enough money and a telephone number for an emergency call. Map out your route to prevent getting lost. During your preparations, it is important to estimate how long it will

There can be little enjoyment in being out in public if you are constantly fretting over your safety. Leave home prepared.

Thorough and sustained precautionary measures are vital to the safety of the disabled.

take. If possible, tell someone where you are going, estimated time you expect to arrive and return, and a phone number where you can be reached. It is also a good idea to inform the place you are going when you are about to leave for your destination. When you make this call, find out about the parking facilities. Is there parking close to the entrance? How well lit is it at night? If the lighting conditions are poor, can you arrange for someone to look out for you? If you feel unsure or unsafe, have someone go with you. If this is not possible, don't go!

If you are traveling by mass transit, follow the same steps, but in addition find out how close to your destination you will be dropped off, and whether someone can meet you at your stop. If there is no one to meet you, or if you cannot go with someone, or if the area is unsafe, don't go! If you are not fearful of going out alone to a strange neighborhood, more power to you. But there are still further considerations.

When traveling always be aware of your environment, and avoid dark and secluded areas. Carry your valuables in a secure place, out of sight. Again, if you can't afford to lose something, don't bring it.

I always use these preparations and precautions before I go anywhere. It's not being obsessive—it's being smart and safe. Having a secure feeling on your way to your destination will keep your mind open to think of more important and pleasant things.

When you have made all your physical preparations for a safe trip and feel confident about it, it is time to explore your mental preparedness. You have prepared for most situations that you can control, but you may still have concerns about those that could arise outside your control. Being concerned is good; not being concerned may result in your making mistakes and perhaps getting hurt.

Dealing with Confrontations

When confronted, realize that you have options other than running. You may be confronted verbally by someone who intends to harass you and eventually rob or assault you. Your initial reactions and mental preparedness will greatly influence the outcome. Since you cannot run, you must rely on your mental skills, and keep a level head. If you can place yourself within eye and ear proximity of a crowd, you can yell out to get attention, which is something attackers don't like. Since most attackers want and expect fear from their victims, they will leave. Your best tactic in confrontational situations is to prevent them. Some of us may be confronted by attackers we know, like work associates, peers, and classmates. How we handle them can also prepare us to deal with attackers on the outside. Being disabled and confronted with verbal abuse by "bullies" is not unusual.

If you are concerned about what to do in a physical confrontation, take classes in self-defense for the disabled, or in the martial arts. You can locate these programs as described above for the visually impaired.

Dealing with Bullies

Who is the bully attacker? What does he want? Where is he usually found? How does he operate? Why does he pick on the disabled? I'll answer this by sharing some of my own experiences and the ways I have dealt with them. (These examples are not meant to indicate that you should do exactly as I did.)

When I was in elementary school most of my activities centered around TV. Socially, most of the kids I hung around with were children of my parents' friends. In school, there were always a few bullies who were constantly harassing me. The school did nothing to stop the teasing, either from ignorance or apathy, and I shied away and took it. Fortunately no physical altercations occurred. But when I reached junior high school, these same bullies became more aggressive. During the first half of the school year the school again did nothing. Neither did I. My brother then told me that I had to confront the ring leader. After seven years of being picked on and doing nothing, I had become fed up. I realized the bullies were all "mouth," and that the only way I would feel good about myself was to deal directly with the problem. So one day I approached the leader and challenged him to a fight. To my amazement and anger, he refused in front of the class. His teasing stopped. That day I learned what kind of person a bully is, and to this day I have not tolerated being demeaned.

When I entered high school, there was another wise guy who tried to put me down. I knew nothing about the martial arts, but I knew it was worth taking a chance, and to his surprise I made him part of the school window. After that show of assertiveness, I never shied away

"The bully" uses intimidation as his primary weapon.

Remember that only a coward would attack an elderly or disabled person.

again. If someone tried to put me down, I told him in front of a crowd that I would not tolerate his remarks.

During my last three years in high school, I was never harassed again. I experienced a new feeling—self-respect. This was not only because I had become involved in sports, but because I had acquired the reputation of never backing down from a confrontation. What I did in school would not necessarily work on the streets, because the person who confronts on the streets is not seeking attention like the bully, but is after something else. But regardless of what kind of a situation you are in, or with whom, whether with a stranger or acquaintance, you should always maintain your self-respect. Without it you will never leave an altercation a winner. If you can feel confident that you did all you could, you will always leave a winner.

Understanding the Assailant

The attackers, for the most part, are people who themselves lack self-esteem, and have a poor self-image. What do they usually want from the disabled? An easy mark, and a way to vent their own frustrations on someone who will not offer resistance. Where are the attacks likely to occur? While the bully usually operates where he is surrounded by his peers, so he can get their attention, the street attacker usually operates in a secluded area. Attackers usually face a disabled person because they first want to instill fear, and believe that you will acquiesce to any of their demands. We look like easy prey to them, and they need to prove something to themselves, mostly their manhood, and they believe we can provide the means.

The most important thing for you to remember, which will help get you through almost anything society can throw at you, is to ask for nothing more than respect, and to accept nothing less.

The following commentary is by Warren D. Williams, who is in his early thirties, and works as a support service coordinator with disabled students. He is confined to a wheelchair.

WARREN'S SELF-DEFENSE STORY

Throughout our history, we have never achieved unconditional social equality. From the time of the Roman Empire, through the Middle Ages to the present day, social inequality has always existed. Some people who are considered unequal in our society will always be treated differently because of their race, sex, ethnic group, or religion. Most tragically, people with physical or mental disabilities are also treated unfairly in society. Here I will define the words "handicapped" and "disabled" as "having natural inequalities."

I happen to have natural inequalities. I have osteogenesis imperfecta, a brittle-bone disorder. During my lifetime I have broken over 150 bones. Osteogenesis imperfecta altered my growth process and I am three feet four inches tall. It has also left me with impaired hearing. It is fair to say my life is hard because of my disabilities, but I absolutely refuse to sit back in my wheelchair and waste it away.

Anyone who wants to survive, whether disabled or not, must learn to adapt to their environment. Some people have inner strength, which does not necessarily make them strong in the physical sense, but in crisis situations it motivates an inner strength. My inner strength generates my adrenaline and stimulates me mentally.

Even now as I write, I can feel it. I sense my subconscious mind telling me that I am strong, invincible, and intelligent. The feeling doesn't tell me I can heal myself, but it does help me adjust to certain situations.

For example, if I drop a pencil on the floor, how can I pick it up? I can either ask someone to pick it up for me, or I can try to pick it up myself. When I am sitting in my wheelchair my arms are too short to reach the floor. Instead of feeling helpless, I figured out a way to pick up things off the floor. I can use my reacher to do it. If I happen to be in a situation where help is unavailable to me, I have to be creative enough to find an alternative solution, such as

Inner strength can be built from reprogramming negative thought patterns.

A flexible, creative mind can overcome all manner of obstacles.

using a coat hanger, broom handle, or kitchen tongs. It is important for anyone with limited mobility to be creative. I have never considered myself handicapped. However, I do consider myself different because of my wheelchair. But having to use a wheelchair has never made me feel inferior or stupid.

Most importantly, having to use a wheelchair never interfered with earning a degree in political science, getting married, and driving a van. My life is very fulfilling. I enjoy such activities as swimming, weight lifting, tennis, and my favorite activity, billiards. Furthermore, I have adopted a new activity, martial arts.

It would be reasonable to say, "Anyone with a brittle-bones disorder has no business participating in a martial arts class." I admit that it can be very dangerous, especially for someone like myself. When I was a teenager, I saw Bruce Lee in Enter the Dragon, and I wanted to take martial arts so badly I could taste it. I could not do so then because my bones and muscles were not strong enough. I can now. Studying martial arts gives me a new sense of self-confidence, and it keeps me in shape. Most importantly, it teaches me how to protect myself against attackers. Unfortunately, being physically disabled has not protected me from violent crime.

About a year ago, I became a victim of such a crime. I was scheduled to take a federal examination at the Federal Building in Newark, New Jersey. The parking guard would not allow me to park in the underground parking lot. So I had to park outside.

I got out of my van and in my wheelchair proceeded to the building. All of a sudden, without warning, two guys jumped me. I said to myself, "This cannot really be happening." There I was, a disabled person in a wheelchair being mugged in broad daylight by two men. They were trying to get my bag that I keep on the back of my wheelchair. I just kept moving, hoping to outmaneuver them, but one grabbed me. Without even thinking about it, I gave that attacker an elbow to the stomach, and a knife chop to the throat. He fell to his knees, but still had enough stamina to fight back. Using my wheelchair as a weapon, I put it in reverse and ran over him. When it was over, there he lay, a pitiful-looking mugger crumpled on the sidewalk. The other attacker saw what I had done to his partner, and decided not to mess with me. I was not injured in the attack. (However, they did take their anger out on my van.)

In conclusion, some people regard me as being handicapped, and as incapable of functioning in society because I have to use a wheelchair to get around. But I accomplish more things sitting in my wheelchair than many people do standing up. I may be different, but I consider myself a human being who deserves to be treated with respect.

RISK REDUCTION FOR THE ELDERLY

All of the recommendations in the chapter on Reducing Your Risk should also be followed if you are older, and many techniques for the disabled should be practiced in the same manner. Confidence is stressed over and over by Vincent Marchetti, active for forty years in martial arts and holder of a seventh-degree black belt in karate, seventh-degree black belt in jujitsu, fifth-degree black belt in Bushido jujitsu, and a second-degree black belt in judo. Elected to the International Karate Hall of Fame, and World Martial Arts Hall of Fame, he has been teaching self-defense to the elderly for over thirty years. Marchetti is also the originator of the "Michi Budo Ryu" system of self-defense, which utilizes three different forms of the martial arts. In addition, Marchetti recommends the following:

✔Carry simple, legal articles you can use as weapons (see pages 00) without hurting yourself.

✔Do not wear heavy chains around your neck. They can be used to choke you.

✔Do not wear pierced hanging earrings. They can be used by an attacker to tear an ear, and then to pull you anywhere he chooses by using the other earring.

✔Do not wear old jewelry, valuable antiques, or heirlooms. Thieves can spot from a distance what is real and what is not. Save these for occasional family affairs, and wear costume jewelry at other times.

Exercise is important for the elderly to maintain flexibility and muscle and bone strength.

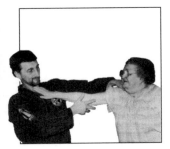

✔Do not carry a purse when going out. Assailants look for this. Carry your money, keys, and credit cards tucked away somewhere. They know it is common for older women to carry a big purse with their keys, wallet, and money. If they grab your purse, they will sometimes take your keys, and meet you back at your apartment or house. If you do not carry one, they will probably look for another victim, rather than have to stop and search you.

✔Carry a cane or walking stick as a matter of habit, and practice how to use it in self-defense. This is a simple precaution for you to take when going out.

✔Whenever possible do not go out alone, or at night.

✔It is very easy to become relaxed when following your normal routines of everyday living. This complacency can produce a lack of awareness, and is what assailants look for and count on.

✔A last important note of caution: It is characteristic of the elderly to walk with their heads down. Yes, they have a lot on their minds: a grandson's birthday, granddaughter's graduation, a host of other family-related matters, health concerns, and financial problems. But this, too, is what muggers look for. They stalk these people in their own neighborhoods, and in their familiar comfort zones, like on the way to the library and senior citizens' clubs, where they are apt to be less aware than they would be in a strange place.

SELF-DEFENSE FOR THE ELDERLY

Although your confidence level is to some degree related to your feelings of physical vulnerability (slowdown in reflexes, loss of sensory sharpness, decrease in strength and stamina), this is by no means the whole story, because everyone, regardless of age, is capable of doing more than they believe they can. For example, your age has nothing to do with your ability to use the heel of your shoe to scrape the shin or instep of an attacker, producing enough pain to make him release his hold on you.

Many older people have come to enjoy becoming involved in self-defense classes where they learn how to do simple things to protect themselves, as for example when being grabbed in various positions. As they see these techniques working for them they begin to believe in them, and they learn that they are capable, not helpless. And this is important because an attacker wants a target, a victim, and not an opponent.

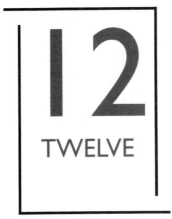

Survival Techniques in Action

TWELVE

A S YOU HAVE READ you have been learning to develop a way of thinking and behaving based upon some newly accepted realities, and a different attitude about your own vulnerability. The following vignettes contain ingredients which represent a range of situations that can occur.

The situations portrayed contain some common elements, because no assault situation is totally unique, though all are complex. An attack can come out of the blue, with no warning, and with an assailant using direct physical force. Some assaults occur so rapidly that there is very little lead-up, and the potential victim cannot see the approaching danger. Such assaults can occur whether or not proper avoidance measures have been taken. Some assault situations unfold slowly, with enough lead-up to allow the potential victim to see the impending danger well in advance of an assault.

Whether you will have the opportunity or ability to break the holding mechanism, if one is operating, and how much of the defensive survival method you will be able to use, will depend upon how fast things are happening. All of these above considerations are included in the following situations.

Note that if you change any one element of an attack situation, the number and kinds of choices you will have and the ways you can behave will also be changed. Thus, each of the following events could have unfolded with a variety of responses by both the potential victim and the assailant. Also, each quarry and each assailant will differ in how they view themselves, others, and the world around them, and their behavior will be determined by these feelings.

Remember, also, that an assailant may stand out in a crowd or may remain obscure in manner and appearance. Most rape victims have described their attackers as having "normal" or ordinary appearances. Just as assailants come in all sizes, shapes, and colors, their mental states and emotions will also vary, and play a dominant role in the course of an assault. In the same way, a potential victim's personality and psychological makeup will also influence his or her behavior during a crime.

The analysis after each situation will discuss how these factors apply. Remember that all kinds of thoughts and feelings occur when a person is in a life-and-death situation.

In each model experience you will see how the situation always dictating the response applies.

You will follow potential victims—who have learned defensive survival techniques—through their thoughts and feelings, through fictitious life-threatening episodes, designed to parallel experiences that real people have encountered. They neither point out correct solutions or courses of action for you to follow, nor do they endorse passive or active resistance, or confrontational versus nonconfrontational behavior. Instead they will teach you to develop your own survival attitude, and create your own edge by learning how others have applied their defensive survival techniques.

A WOMAN HELD CAPTIVE IN HER CAR

It was a beautiful Saturday morning, warm and sunny, so I decided to get an early start.

I drove to the supermarket. The parking lot was unusually full so I drove around for a while and finally gave up trying to find a space close to the store. I parked farther away from the entrance than I preferred, especially when I had so much to buy. Oh well, I thought, no big deal! As I got out of the car all I could think of was getting in and out of the market as fast as possible. I noticed a tall, lanky man who was walking behind me, and who followed me into the store. I thought nothing

> There is no such thing as right or wrong forms of resistance, simply more or less effective ways of dealing with each situation.

Leave your worries at home. When out in public focus on your surroundings and listen to your intuition.

more about it at the time, nor of his presence near me frequently, partly because he was so ordinary-looking.

At the check-out counter, I remember him looking at me, but did not connect this to any possible danger.

With my cart full, I quickly left the store and proceeded to my car. I was in a hurry, walking fast, and looking only for where I had parked it. I was unaware that a would-be assailant was not far behind me. Before opening the tailgate, I gave my usual quick glance around and saw no one, except a group of teenagers laughing and having fun a little behind and to my left. I loaded the packages into the car, closed the tailgate, looked around again quickly, walked to the driver's door, unlocked it, and swung it open.

It was too late. I had not seen him follow me and lose himself behind the crowd of teenagers. He was on me in a flash. I no sooner had my door open than I felt myself being pushed into the car from behind. In an instant I found myself on the passenger side, and he was behind the wheel pointing an opened switchblade at my stomach. I was able to get a clear look at him. He was tall, as ordinary-looking as anyone else, and dressed in slacks, a sport jacket, and clean-shaven.

I was numb. I knew this was happening to me and yet I couldn't believe it. I was dazed, and couldn't think. Two minutes ago I was light-hearted and carefree, looking forward to the evening. Now the only thing on my mind was what was going to happen to me.

Then he spoke. "Do exactly what I say and you won't get hurt." Looking at his long body, all of a sudden I felt shorter than I actually was, and very vulnerable. His size intimidated me so much that for a few seconds I began to wonder if I was ever going to get out of this alive.

The drive to our initial destination seemed like an eternity, but it was only a few blocks to a deserted area where he stopped the car. He grabbed my wrist and got out of the car, pulling me with him. Then he walked me around to the passenger side and said, "Get behind the wheel," and got in next to me.

I now realized that I was a captive in my own car, and unaware of my attacker's plan. I was pretty sure at this point that I was going to be raped, because he had not attempted a mugging, and he was taking me somewhere. The thought of rape sent chills through my body. I decided I must somehow escape.

I kept silent so that I wouldn't say something that might anger him, until I could get some idea of his personality. My mind was going double-time. He had not tried to hurt me so far, I thought. Even the way he grabbed my arm and maneuvered me to the other side of the car was not done roughly or brutally. But still, he had that knife always ready to use. My confusion mounted.

I began to try and use defensive survival psychology and the F.I.T. method as best I could. I *focused* on details and the conditions through which I was driving. Out of the corner of my eye I noticed that he was no longer holding the knife quite so tightly nor was he pointing it in my direction. He seemed more intent on where we were going.

I was also very interested in where we were going because I had made the decision not to allow myself to be raped, even if I had to fight like hell. My first plan was to try and escape. But how? I hadn't the slightest idea of where to start. He has a knife, and he is a man, I thought. All I have is a steering wheel in my hand. That's it! All of a sudden it hit me. I am in control of a heavy piece of powerful machinery. He was only in control of me, or so he thought. He did not know my intentions or plans, either.

At that moment, I made a conscious decision to use the car as my weapon and means of escape. Because I had decided to do something concrete to try and take control, I began to feel just a little more composed. I thought of the relaxation and *imagery* exercises I had been practicing, and wondered how well I could manage to use them under such stress and fear. What have I got to lose? I thought.

I *focused* more intently on the surroundings and streets we were traveling, looking desperately for some familiar areas. I wondered which would be better, running into a storefront to attract people or hitting a police car. Which would offer me a better chance to get away? Would people come to my assistance? What if they didn't? Question after question went through my mind. At the same time, I was trying to *isolate* any other danger signs that could be reasons not to go through with either plan. I couldn't find any. My attacker did not seem suspicious of me, and my gut feeling said, "Go for it."

In a hostage or kidnapping situation keep yourself alert to lapses in your assailant's attention or concentration.

Appearances are often deceptive. Don't be fooled by smart clothes and a clean-shaven face.

I began to get myself ready, still not knowing exactly what I was going to do, but sure I was going to do something. I tried to become aware of my *feelings*. I knew I was terrified but I also felt my commitment to escape.

I kept up the relaxation exercise. My heart was not thumping quite so hard, and I was able to start thinking of the *technique* I should use.

Now was the time to use the *imagery* skills I had been developing. I imagined myself going through the motions, step by step. I concentrated on my surroundings, but did not let myself get caught up with my attacker or his weapon. I began to *imagine* my escape as if it were happening before my eyes. I searched and searched for the right store, or a police car. But everything was unfamiliar, and the area sparsely populated. Meanwhile, I knew time was passing and we would soon be reaching my attacker's destination. And then I saw the green lights far ahead on the front of a building, and I knew exactly where we were.

Everything started to fall into place, in a matter of seconds. I knew I was wearing my seat belt and that my assailant was not. I *thought* now is the time! I floored the accelerator pedal and the car shot off from forty-five miles per hour to fifty-five to sixty-five. Then I hit the brakes hard with all my might. As the car came to an abrupt halt, he went flying into the dash, hitting his head on the windshield. I quickly unbuckled my seatbelt, opened the door, and went flying into Engine Company 711. It was over.

Survival Skills Analysis

Could this victim have prevented herself from becoming a captive? The answer is a definite "Yes." There were four separate points at which she could have escaped.

✔ *Had she been more focused on her surroundings and the unfolding events, her intuition might have told her to be somewhat suspicious, and more alert and careful. Noticing him enter the store behind her, and shopping all this time in close proximity to her, should have made her consider the possibility of danger.*

✔ *The next missed opportunity was when she left the store, and her assailant would still have been visible to her. Not until he used the group of teenagers for his cover did he become hidden.*

✔*Another opportunity was when she reached her car, but she only glanced around quickly when opening the tailgate, and then when she closed it. If she had been more observant she might have noticed him making his moves, since he had to be closing in on her to get to her in time when she opened the car door.*

✔*Her last missed opportunity was when she opened the door and her assailant was almost next to her. She had never isolated any advance signs of danger. If her attacker had been unkempt, with long disheveled hair, or dressed in boots and leather adorned with spiked bracelets and chains, she would almost certainly have taken notice of him early on and perhaps been more careful. And if she had not been so preoccupied, she might not have stood out as being a "good" prospect for an assault.*

This assailant was not verbally abusive, or overwhelmingly hostile. He gave the impression that he was there to do what he "must," and the faster and more easily this could be accomplished with a minimum of force and violence, the better. This, of course, was to her advantage.

A self-assured and well-organized person, with an ability to act decisively, she was able to make and carry out the decision to escape, to *focus* on the subtleties of what was taking place between her assailant and herself, and most important, to make a split-second decision to abandon a failing strategy and pursue something else.

A WOMAN ATTACKED IN HER SUBURBAN HOME

My husband was away on a business trip, and I did not expect him home until mid-morning.

When the doorbell rang, at eight-fifteen, I couldn't imagine who it could be at that hour. I looked through the peephole and saw a man with his back towards me. He had on a short jacket like most delivery men wear. I asked "Who is it?" A voice replied, "Special delivery, ma'am." I couldn't see if he had a package, since he was not facing me. When I looked out of the window I didn't see a truck or any other vehicle nearby. I remember thinking that was kind of peculiar. But as deliveries of all kinds are very common in my neighborhood I didn't dwell

Always ask for identification from delivery people. If you are not expecting anything, be especially cautious.

on it. For a split-second I felt a reluctance to open the door. I asked "Can you leave it on the front stoop?" "'Fraid not ma'am. I need your signature."

As soon as I unlocked the door, it swung open with such force that it threw me backwards, almost knocking me off my feet. There, facing me, knife in hand, was this tall, broadly built man. He appeared to be in his twenties, was unshaven, dressed in jeans and sneakers. His eyes were glassy. The first thing I thought was that he was on drugs.

"Take it easy, and you won't get hurt," were his first words.

Hardly able to speak, I stammered, "What do you want?"

"You are alone, aren't you?" I couldn't get the words out. "Aren't you?" he asked, louder, and more menacing, thrusting the knife forward in a threatening way.

"Yes, yes," I stammered.

He seemed satisfied and lowered his knife slightly. He looked around, and indicated to me by motioning with his knife to walk ahead of him.

I walked from room to room. When we got to the bedroom he stopped. This is it, I thought.

If I was fearful before, I was now in an all-out state of panic, and could think of nothing but the word "rape."

But he made no move towards me. Instead, he opened the drawers of my husband's bureau and my dresser and started rummaging through them, taking some jewelry, and stuffing it into his pockets. He seemed agitated.

"Don't you have any money around?"

He saw my purse and grabbed it. I only had a few dollars and was intending to go to the bank that day.

"I need more!" he said angrily.

I was a little calmer now since I felt he wasn't going to rape me, and I began to think of some strategies. "I could write you a check," I blurted out. "Here, look. You could have all this money." I showed him the balance in the checking account.

He was suspicious, and didn't want to give his name. I told him I could make it out to cash. I thought of putting a note on the back of the check saying, GET HELP. CALL POLICE. I knew the bank teller would have to turn over the check to look for my signature.

But I discarded the idea as too risky. I quickly tore a check out of the book, made it out to "Cash" for the entire balance in the account, and handed it to him. I could see he was still not convinced, but he took it.

"You can take it to any bank. Believe me. They'll cash it with no questions asked. Will you go now?" I begged.

But he said, "Oh, I don't know. Maybe I'll stick around a while and keep you company. A nice lady like you shouldn't be alone." He came closer and began stroking my hair. I had no doubt then that he was going to rape me. Again I was in a panic. Everything had changed, and I couldn't think clearly, though I knew I had to.

He asked, "You aren't expecting anyone, are you?" I remembered a friend was going to stop by to return something she had borrowed. She knew I would be home. But I was pretty sure she wouldn't suspect anything was wrong. She would probably think I'd forgotten she was coming.

If my husband's plane was on time he could be home before very long.

"Well?" my attacker asked. There was an urgency in his voice.

"No, no, of course not," I said.

"Good. We don't want any interruptions, do we? I hope your husband isn't in the habit of coming home for anything. I'd hate to have to hurt him." As he said this, he smiled, waving the knife around.

Oh, my God, I thought. If he walks in, he may be killed. I knew I couldn't stall for time. Every moment counted, but what was I to do? Then the unexpected happened. My attacker demanded food!

He walked into the kitchen and sat down at the kitchen table. I went over to the cupboard to start looking for something to make. As soon as I opened the cabinets, I spotted the hot pepper from Mexico. We had never used it because it was so strong. I knew exactly what I was going to do: dump the whole container in the pan of food.

I was now able to think a little more clearly. I got out the food and pots, and went to work. At the same time, I knew I had to gain control of myself enough to make my plan work, and to recognize everything I was *feeling*. I realized how scared I was, and wondered if I could carry out my plan. While standing at the stove I began to go through my relaxation exercise, and then I was able to start *imagining* the *technique* I would use. While I was preparing his meal, I went through everything, step by step, over and over, ending with the safety and survival *imagery*.

Between 1981 and 1991 the ratio of homicide rates between the U.S. and Canada, based upon 100,000 inhabitants, was 3.4 : 1.

Practice spontaneity. When in different locales make a quick mental inventory of potential defensive weapons.

When I brought over his plate of food he grabbed my arm and said, "You are going to eat with me, right?"

"Sure," I replied. "Take a taste and see if it's OK."

As I turned back to the stove, he jumped up from the chair, grabbing his throat and yelling. "Now" I *thought* and grasped the handle of the big heavy pot of boiling water, like it was a baseball bat, and swung it at his face, making sure I was out of the line of fire. He screamed, as his arms went upwards. I swung the pot again with all my might and hit him squarely on the forehead. I did not stop to look, but ran as fast as I could out the front door, still holding the pot. I kept on running, and then I saw my mailman.

"Help me!" I screamed. "There's a man in my house!"

The mailman quickly took my arm and led me to his mail truck. He wanted to drive me to the police station, but I was worried my husband might come home to find this injured man in the house. He might be killed. We called the police from a neighbor's house. I suggested that we park where we could watch for my husband and warn him.

In just a few minutes the block was filled with police cars and the house was surrounded. The robber had already fled, but as the police had a good description of him, he was shortly apprehended.

Survival Skills Analysis

What mistakes did this victim make and what did she do correctly?

✔Without opening the door she should have asked the man several things: to tell her the name of the delivery service, to hold up his ID to the peephole, to say who the delivery was for, and to hold the package up so that she could read the address label.

✔Her intuition provided warnings which she did not heed. She could not see a vehicle near the house, and she questioned the early hour for delivery people to be on the road. She had also felt some hesitation about opening the door.

When the man refused to leave the package, she could have told him to put the slip requiring her signature under the door or in the mailbox for him to pick up later or when he was in the area again. Most delivery people will do this.

✔ *She could also have called out loudly something like, "Marty, will you see who it is? I'm busy," and waited to see what he would do.*

✔ *Though she had been focusing on all the right things, and had certainly isolated some significant danger signs, she did not make proper use of either this information or of her intuition.*

✔ *When her assailant pushed open the door, forcing her backwards, she could have immediately turned and run for the house's back door, grabbing anything she could get her hands on to throw in his way, and knocking over furniture as she ran to slow him down. Once outside, she could have screamed to attract attention, and run to a neighbor. Doing this would have broken the holding mechanism.*

Once he was in the house, she handled herself well. She made no wrong moves, nor did she say anything to escalate the situation.

✔ *Since she had very little cash on hand, it was a clever move to try to encourage him to go to the bank with her check, in the hope that his need for money would be greater than his need to rape (if, indeed, this was part of his plan).*

✔ *Her decision not to tell her attacker about a friend dropping by and that her husband was coming home was a gamble. If she had told him, he might have been scared off and decided to quickly get away. But he might also have become angry and not have believed her, thinking she was merely trying to scare him off. In any case, she had reason to be afraid that he would wait for her husband and harm him, since he had already threatened to do so.*

✔ *Her use of the hot pepper in his food to disable him enough for her to throw the scalding water on his face proved an effective tactic. She was also right to follow this with a strike to his head using the heavy pot, because she had remembered two things: someone under the influence of drugs can withstand an inordinate amount of pain, and may be able to fight even with broken limbs or bullet wounds. She also remembered that the eyes are one of the most vulnerable and effective parts of the body to attack.*

The more quickly you can break the holding mechanism, the greater your chances of escaping unharmed.

> ✔Immediately removing herself from the house, finding help, having the mailman watch for her husband to warn him not to enter the house, and calling the police, in that order, were all correct moves.

She did all the right things during the assault to create her edge, but all the wrong ones before it.

A WOMAN FOLLOWED INTO HER GARAGE

This was one of those days I was thankful that my husband had convinced me to let him install one of those automatic garage door openers. The rain was coming down so heavily my wipers could barely clear the windshield enough to see. As I pulled into the garage, I thought I caught a fleeting glimpse of someone trying to sneak inside behind the car before the door closed completely. I argued with myself that I was being silly, but nevertheless felt hesitant in getting out of the car. The thought crossed my mind to just start the car again, open the garage door and back out. Before I could think any further or come to any decision, I saw him. He was walking towards the front of the car and grinning. I immediately pressed the transmitter to open the door but nothing happened. Sure enough, I saw the plug had been disconnected. I was in a state of sheer panic. Fortunately, my doors were all locked, but I was still a prisoner in my own car.

There he stood, still grinning. He was of medium height, thin, unshaven, had long hair, and was dressed in a sweater, sweat pants, sneakers and a baseball cap. He didn't seem to be in a hurry to get at me. It was like he was enjoying watching me squirm. This made me feel angry as well as fearful, and I wished I had some way to hurt him. My anger and desire to get at him were so intense, I think they helped me concentrate on a way of escaping. I felt my heart pounding. I had to calm down. I did the relaxation and imagery exercises as best I could.

I thought of running him down, but he stayed away from the front of the car, and I knew if I got out of the car, I wouldn't stand a chance of escaping. I felt so helpless, I couldn't attract attention. I thought of leaning on the horn, but who would be concerned about a horn being sounded in a garage? Who would even know where it was coming from?

Don't advertise yourself as a tourist or vacationer. Thieves know holiday makers have plenty of money.

I focused on the garage as I never had before, seeing things I was never really aware of, but I quickly realized that the car was my only solution. Suddenly he grabbed a tire iron from the wall, and came straight at the windshield waving it.

Quickly, I hit the horn. The sudden blast jolted him to the point where he stopped in his tracks, but only for a split-second. It gave me time enough to start the engine, shift into reverse and floor the accelerator. The car crashed back into the door, but it didn't go through. I quickly put it into drive, pulled forward all the way to the front wall, and then reversed it again. The weakened door gave way and out I went amid a mass of splintering wood.

The loud crash, of course, attracted some neighbors' attention. Out of the garage ran my assailant, and he kept on running. I was so mad, I considered going after him with the car, but I decided to leave that job for the police.

Survival Skills Analysis

This woman missed her only opportunity to prevent herself from becoming a captive. The moment she first felt something might be wrong, when she thought someone had followed her into the garage, she should have immediately backed out onto the street a safe distance away. She could then have sounded her horn to attract attention.

✔When the situation had escalated to the next stage, she had limited options, but what she had, she used well. Blasting the horn as a distraction to give her a few more seconds to act was a good decision.

✔Her one viable choice was to use the car exactly as she did.

A COUPLE ATTACKED IN THEIR HOME

My wife, retired like myself, was upstairs taking a nap and I had dozed off in the den. I awakened with a start when I thought I heard a noise in the basement. I got up to investigate, and as I opened the basement door I came face to face with a small but menacing-looking man dressed in a sweater, corduroy pants, and an old torn army jacket.

Home alarms can now be purchased and installed at a very reasonable cost.

If you sense you are in danger, try not to isolate yourself. Make sure you go to, or stay with, other people.

We were both surprised, and stood staring at each other, me on the top landing of the stairs, and he, one or two steps below. I had a sudden urge to push him backwards. He would have fallen down fourteen steps. In my moment of hesitation, he pulled out a huge switchblade and pointed it at my chest. I backed up.

"All I want is your money and jewelry." I gave him my wallet.

"Is this all you got? Don't you have any more? What about jewelry?" He was very edgy. I was also afraid he might go up to the bedroom to search. Question after question raced through my head. What if my wife wakes up and hears voices? Suppose she calls down to me? I didn't know what to do next. I did know that I had to calm down if I was going to be able to think of a way to get both of us out of this. As I walked from room to room with him close behind me, I did some relaxation and *imagery* procedures. I *imagined* Mary in bed, and the assailant walking up the stairs and barging in on her, and all the terrible things that could happen. And this was how an idea came to me. I thought for a moment and said, "Look, my wife is very sick." I said. "She has a bad heart and is in bed. If she sees you, the shock could kill her. Let me go upstairs and get you what you want, and you wait here."

He hesitated, not sure I was telling the truth, but I urged him to go see for himself.

"You go first," he said.

I had to be convincing so I *imagined* myself walking up the stairs very slowly with him following, and then motioning for him to stay quiet while I looked into the room. I did everything just as I had rehearsed it in my mind. We walked up the stairs and looked in at my wife sleeping, or so it appeared. For the first time, I began feeling less scared and more in control. To get him away from the bedroom, I turned back down the stairs knowing he would follow me to make sure I wasn't up to something. I hoped my wife was awake and had heard what was going on.

He said, "OK, so you convinced me. Now go back up and get me that money and jewelry. No tricks, or you'll both be sorry."

I returned to the bedroom. My wife was awake, as I had suspected. She pointed to the phone and mouthed the words, "I called the police." I nodded, grabbed some cash and rings and went down.

"Here," I said, to him, "This is everything." He took the money and jewelry, and ran out of the house. But he did not get far, because he was quickly surrounded by several police cars.

My wife told me that she had heard what was happening downstairs and had called the police. When she described the circumstances to them, they told her to go back to bed, and pretend she was asleep in case the assailant decided to return to the bedroom.

Survival Skills Analysis

The victim in this situation had very few options. If he had tried to escape, it would have meant leaving his wife alone with the assailant. The other choice of waking her, and then both trying an escape could have resulted in harm to either or both of them.

✔ *He had one sure opportunity which he had missed: when he and the assailant came to face to face. If he had followed through on his sudden urge to push his assailant backwards down the steps, the holding mechanism would have been broken.*

✔ *His attempt to convince the intruder to believe his story about his wife without investigating further was an appropriate gamble under the circumstances.*

A WOMAN AVOIDING ASSAULT IN A PARKING LOT

When I park in a mall, I always make it a point to choose a space which is easily accessible and close to the stores. This is what I had done that day. After I was through shopping, I walked to my car taking all the precautions I had learned as I approached it. As I *focused* on my surroundings, everything looked clear. Then I noticed the van. It had not been there before, and was now parked next to my car with its side door parallel to my driver's side. My heart began to race though there was really no need for alarm. I wasn't in any danger, yet a feeling had really upset me. Somehow I was *feeling* that I was coming very close to a dangerous situation.

In the U.S. the average person is now about twice as likely to be murdered as twenty-five years ago.

> If something doesn't "feel" right, it probably isn't.

I immediately turned and walked back into the mall. There I found a quiet spot and went through a relaxation exercise. As soon as I had calmed down I located a security guard. Apologetic and somewhat embarrassed, I asked him to walk me to my car, explaining about the van parked beside it.

I opened the door opposite the driver's side while the guard stood beside me. I thanked him, locked the door, slid over behind the wheel, and drove away. But then something made me stop a distance away and watch the van for a few minutes. Sure enough, it moved and pulled into a space next to a car that a woman had just gotten out of. I located another security guard and told him what had happened. He radioed the police, and I left.

Survival Skills Analysis

This woman is to be commended on the manner in which she kept *focused* on her immediate surroundings, and *isolated* the significant potential danger signs.

✔ *Her strategy of having a security guard (or storekeeper) accompany her to her car was perfect.*

✔ *But her follow-up actions were also important. Her intuition told her more danger was lurking for someone else. So, knowing she was safe, she acted to help ensure the safety of others.*

AN ATTEMPTED ACQUAINTANCE RAPE

When my friend called to invite me and my husband over for bridge, I told her he was away overnight, so bridge was out. But she urged me to come over anyway, and I accepted. She added that her husband would pick me up on his way from work, and also drive me back at the end of the evening.

Not long after I got to their house, the front doorbell rang, and the host greeted a tall, thin, good-looking younger man, and ushered him inside. He was introduced as his company's new accountant, who had recently graduated with very high marks.

As the evening wore on, I started to feel uncomfortable. I frequently caught glimpses of him looking at me, but decided he just thought I was attractive and that there was nothing more to it. It did unnerve me a bit, though.

When the evening was drawing to an end, and the host was putting on his coat to take me home, the young man asked him where he was going, and when he explained I needed a ride home, quickly replied that he could drive me as he needed to stop at his office on the way.

I was about to interrupt and just say outright that I would prefer my friend to take me, when he said, "It's OK, it will save me a trip." I had the same unnerving feeling again, but was also feeling a little guilty about making someone go out just to drive me home. So I got into this man's car and we drove to his office. As he parked the car, he said, "Why don't you come in for a moment. I don't want you to sit here alone so late at night." This took me completely by surprise, for I had planned to wait for him in the car. He got out and came around to my side. When I made no attempt to move, he gently but firmly took me by the arm, coaxing me out of the car, saying, "I won't be long." I felt an urgent need to pull my arm away and tell him I preferred to wait, but I didn't, thinking I was probably overreacting.

Once in the office, he made some gestures as if he was looking for his papers, then he went to the liquor cabinet, took out some glasses and a bottle. At that point, I knew trouble was brewing. I felt scared but determined not to let him touch me.

When he offered me a drink, I refused and said "I want to go now." But he said, "Oh, loosen up! I'm sure you know you're a very attractive lady." Then he poured two huge drinks, motioned me to take one, and downed the other all at once. I refused, and started to walk towards the door, but before I knew it, he was blocking the door, saying, "C'mon, you're not going to fight me now, are you?"

Things were happening so fast, the only thing I could think of was keeping him from getting to me. I quickly *focused* on the room, scanning it as quickly as possible, while watching him.

He was still standing with his back towards the door. I quickly placed myself with the desk between us. It was one of those oversized executive ones, with an overhang on all three sides. I knew he wouldn't

Always carry enough cash so that, if the need arises, you can take a cab home.

be able to vault over it very easily, especially in his condition. The alcohol was beginning to slow him up, his speech was starting to slur, he was unsteady and uncoordinated.

He was getting mad. He poured himself another drink, saying, "Damn you, you'll be sorry for this!"

I had never seen such a fast personality change. His eyes were wide open and glassy, and his fists clenched. I had noticed that the door to the adjoining office was open. I thought of trying to make my way into it and locking the door, but I didn't know how I was going to get away to do it. I kept *focusing* on every object around me.

Meanwhile, he slowly started to circle the desk. As he reached one end, there was only the big high-back swivel chair between us. The other office was directly behind me. With my foot I pushed the chair straight at him. He was startled and thrown slightly backwards, but I knew that wouldn't slow him enough to give me time to get through the door, so I grabbed the phone with both hands and hurled it. I ran into the office and locked the door. But now I was trapped. While he pounded on the door shouting obscenities, I quickly phoned my friends and told them what was happening. Before they could speak I heard the phone go dead.

"Pretty smart, but that won't help you!" he yelled, sounding completely out of control. "You can't go anywhere, and as soon as I find the key, you're dead!"

I had to get myself out of my panic state. I started working on this with my relaxation and *imagery* exercises. He was yelling so loudly I couldn't finish them, but I became composed enough to start thinking of how to protect myself. I now feared for my life.

I began to *focus* on the room and everything in it. The office was big and sumptuous. There was a closet on one side and a small washroom off to the back, but I couldn't hide in either of them. I could find nothing to use as a weapon. Any minute I expected to hear the key in the door.

Then I noticed the tall, thin halogen floor lamp in the corner. It reminded me of a barbell. If only I could make him lunge at me in the dark, and trip over the lamp. I decided on the *technique* I would use and began to *imagine* everything as if it were happening right before my eyes.

I unplugged the lamp and laid it horizontally across the floor about four feet in front of the door. The pole was just high enough so his foot would get caught under it as he rushed at me. The desk was directly ahead as you entered the room. I moved the two chairs obstructing it and turned out the lights, figuring it would take his eyes a few seconds to adjust to the dark. I stood in hiding to one side of the door and waited.

I soon heard the key in the lock. He was calling me names, muttering and threatening. As he lunged into the room he tripped over the lamp pole. Across the room and over the desk he went. Instantly, I was out of the office, slamming the door closed behind me, and running down the corridor.

My friends and the police all arrived together, and he was quickly apprehended. I was surprised to see all of them. It seems they had heard just enough of my telephone plea for help before my attacker had pulled out the phone line.

Survival Skills Analysis

What did this victim do wrong? Just about everything. Her gut feelings were giving her constant warnings, but she ignored them all. She had several opportunities to get away and break the holding mechanism before becoming a victim. Her uncomfortable feeling about her assailant while playing cards was the beginning of the long line of intuitive warnings.

✔ *The first time she could have acted upon her intuition was when he offered to drive her home. She had felt like interrupting, but her host's response and her feelings of guilt stopped her. She could have asked to speak to her host alone and then told him of her reluctance to go with this man.*

✔ *The next opportunity came when her assailant asked her to accompany him up to the office: she could have jumped out of the car and run.*

✔ *Once they were in the office, events were moving slowly enough at the very beginning for her to have run out of the door and to keep on going. But by the time the situation had escalated, escape became impossible.*

It was fortunate that she was ingenious enough to formulate a strategy which worked for her.

> *No matter what the outcome of an assault or potential assault, the victim suffers trauma.*

PREVENTING AN ATTACK WHILE DRIVING

The relatively low cost and availability of cellular phones these days makes them a wise investment for solo drivers.

When I left the meeting I was tired, but did not allow my fatigue to divert my attention from the rearview mirror. I always make a habit of watching all other cars around me. I had only traveled a few miles when I suspected I was being followed. To confirm my suspicions I made a few zigzag turns to see if the car behind would follow. It did. The danger signs were clearly evident.

I was *feeling* shaken and scared. Everything I had read and heard at safety lectures started to go through my head, all jumbled and mixed up. I knew I had to calm down, so I went through a relaxation exercise I had been using routinely.

I was able to think a little more clearly now. I knew I should stay on busy, well-lighted roads, and find a police station. Fortunately, I was in a familiar neighborhood. I also knew it was important to note the car's description and, if possible, the license plates.

I started to *imagine* what I would do if I could get to the station, and the *technique* I would use. I was hoping my would-be assailants would not make their move before I could get to my destination, a few miles away. Unfortunately, they did.

When I stopped for a traffic light they pulled up next to me. I looked straight ahead, not letting on that I was aware of them. As the light changed, they stayed on my left, abreast of me. I was about half a mile from the police station. I *thought*, and realized I dared not wait. I leaned on the horn, sounding it in long bursts, and sped up. They must have been startled, and began to slow down slightly. A block from the station, I sounded the horn steadily, flashing my high and low beams. As I pulled up, some police officers were already coming out to investigate. The car was no longer in sight. I gave the police all the information, and they assured me they would investigate.

The officers wanted to escort me home, but I was afraid the men might be waiting nearby to see where I lived. The police suggested that we wait to see if their car would be located, since it could not have traveled very far. Sure enough, within fifteen minutes, it was located and the two men were in custody.

Survival Skills Analysis

This woman was *focused* on her surroundings from the start, and rapidly *isolated* the relevant danger signs. She was also aware of her *feelings* and recognized the need to gain emotional control.

✔ The strategy she chose to gain an edge was effective, and her use of imagery helped her carry out the techniques (zigzagging, use of the horn) correctly.

✔ She correctly chose to make her move earlier than she had planned. When danger appeared imminent, she mobilized herself to think and act fast. (Sounding the horn at that time caught the assailants off guard, and jarred them long enough for her to effect her escape.)

✔ She was wise not to proceed to her house right away, and to wait and see if the potential assailants would be apprehended.

✔ Staying on busy, well-lit streets kept her followers from using force, permitting her to remain essentially in control of what was happening.

AN ATTEMPTED ARMED ASSAULT ON THE SUBWAY

I left the office with one of our new law clerks. He asked which way I was going, and I said I was catching a bus or cab. He asked me to ride part way with him because he wanted to discuss some aspects of the trial, and said that he was taking the subway. I was reluctant, and said that I didn't ride the subway if at all possible. He told me I was foolish and a "worry-wart," and that he would be riding most of the way with me. I felt embarrassed and guilty for showing anxiety to this young macho kid. Here I was, the big boss-man showing fear and vulnerability to the new trainee. So, I found myself walking towards the subway.

We boarded the train and the car was not crowded. At one end there were some parents and children; at the other end a few adults of various ages. My companion walked towards a seat in the middle area where it was quieter. I would have preferred to sit nearer to other people, but I

There are times where it may be in your best interest to be pulled over for speeding or haphazard driving.

said nothing. We spoke for a while, and then his stop approached, and he got off.

As he was leaving the car, one new passenger got on. He was about twenty-two, tall and robust, and wearing leather, chains, a bandanna, and boots. My intuition told me that he could spell trouble and I had a sudden urge to get out.

He walked in slowly, looked around, and went towards the end of the car where the adults were sitting. He sat there for a while, frequently looking at me. He grinned and, taking a switchblade from his boot, began opening and closing it. I knew it was just a matter of time before I was in big trouble.

As I returned the papers I had been reading to my attaché case, my hand came upon a spray canister of mace. I had completely forgotten it was there. I wondered if it even worked, since it was very old, and I was hesitant to rely on it.

Before I could think of a plan, I had to deal with the near panic state I was in. I went through my relaxation and *imagery* exercises, and found myself feeling better, and *focusing* on everything around me. I knew running through the cars would be futile since he was bigger, younger, and probably faster than me. And I was pretty sure I could not depend on help from anyone there.

I noticed my *feelings*, how scared I was, and wondered if I could possibly carry out what I was thinking—to fiercely thrust my attaché case into his groin, and then spray him with the mace, if he tried to assault me. I had never committed a violent or physically aggressive act against anyone.

I *imagined* exactly what I would do if he came at me, the *technique* I would use, and the steps that would follow. I had to get in touch with my *feelings*, and overcome any anxiety that might cause me to hesitate.

He got out of his seat and sauntered in my direction, moving slowly and trying to create as much fear as possible by tossing the opened knife from one hand to the other. I kept watching him out of the corner of my eye, giving him no indication that I was aware of what he was doing. I tightened my grip on my attaché case and, as he got closer, I waited for the right moment. When I *thought*, "now", I thrust the corner of the case hard into his groin. He screamed and dropped to his knees. To make doubly sure he was disabled, I sprayed the mace directly into his

Certain types of areas are more likely to harbor certain criminal elements.

eyes. He screamed again. He was trying to get up to grab me but was unable to see. The other passengers sat motionless, as if hypnotized. I ran through the cars to the last one, wondering what would happen next. I waited, fearful that he would still come after me. The train finally reached a station, and I got out, looking all around. Four cars down, I saw a few men escorting my assailant on to the platform.

I did not wait to see what was going to happen next, and went up the stairs to the street. Once there, I hailed a cab to take me home.

Survival Skills Analysis

None of this had to happen. This man's biggest, most obvious mistake was putting his self-image before his safety, and giving priority to how his new law clerk would view him. This prevented him from heeding his intuition.

✔ *Even after this major error, he might still have prevented the rest from occurring, but he again permitted his companion to call the shots when his gut feeling was to sit near other people and not in isolation.*

✔ *His final error was when he saw his would-be assailant enter the train and he ignored how he felt at that moment. Even after having isolated the danger signs, and having bad intuitive feelings, he did nothing. At this point, he had one last chance to move to another car or dart out of the car before the door closed.*

✔ *His choice of a strategy was appropriate. He used his attaché case effectively, and his decision to follow up with the mace also proved correct. Had he used the mace first and it did not work, he would not have had a second chance.*

A WOMAN MUGGED ON THE STREET

It was just about dark when I finished a report after working overtime at the office. Everyone had already left and I was dead tired. The building was almost empty and I felt queasy walking down the long corridor to the elevator. The clicking of my heels on the hard floor echoed and bounced off the walls. That also was a little eerie.

The bus stop was only a few blocks away, and I was relieved to be

> The U.S. Bureau of Justice Statistics says that about two-thirds of crimes are not reported to the police.

Police reporting procedure errors means an undercounting of victims by about 60 to 70 percent.

out of that building. As I approached the waiting area, I was thinking about the pot roast in the refrigerator, and whether my husband would have remembered to prepare the vegetables.

There was no one waiting for the bus, which was taking a long time to come. I opened my purse to see what change I had, but it was too dim to see, so I walked towards the street light. At that moment a firm hand grabbed my arm, and I found myself staring at a long, shiny knife blade.

"Give me all your money, and I won't hurt you. All I want is your money. Move around the corner, out of sight," he said, pushing my arm so my body moved in the direction he was indicating. I couldn't see him too clearly in the shadows. He was wearing a knitted hat pulled down over his ears, and a short heavy jacket. He was about my height.

I couldn't get control of my thoughts and *feelings*. Even though he said he wouldn't hurt me, I didn't know whether to believe him. I thought of screaming to attract attention, but didn't know if I was able to. While he was pushing me, I thought of breaking loose and running, but I was too scared. The last thing I wanted to do was to try to defend myself.

I knew I had to calm down if I was to survive. I began my relaxation and breathing exercise during the short time we were walking.

I was able to *focus* on my surroundings a little better now, and tried to look for people or cars that might help in my escape, though I wasn't sure how I was going to go about it. I saw a vagrant half a block away who could barely keep his balance he was so full of alcohol. That gave me an idea. I would use a diversion to distract my attacker and then run. I quickly *imagined* the *technique* I was going to use, and how and when I was going to act.

When we'd reached the corner, he demanded my money. I trembled and fumbled with my purse, trying to stall for as much time as possible.

"Please, please," I begged. "I'll give you everything, just be patient." I trembled more.

He had lowered his knife, and was concentrating on my purse, not even looking at my face. I could see he was getting impatient, and was afraid he would grab the purse from me, or even hit me, and then my whole plan would fail.

Just then I saw some cars coming into view. I *thought* for a moment, dropped my purse to distract him, and ran in front of them screaming,

"Help, police!" The cars had now passed between my attacker and me, and I kept on running and yelling. As I got to the other side of the street, a delivery truck stopped, and I told the driver what had happened. He had a mobile radio in the truck, and quickly called for help. There was no sign of my attacker, but the driver waited until the police arrived just to make sure I would be safe.

Survival Skills Analysis

Events worked out in this woman's favor because her assailant achieved his main goal of obtaining her purse, and because she was able to get away and attract attention to herself.

✔ *She was correct in giving up her personal possessions, and waiting for the right opportunity to make her escape.*

✔ *She need not, however, have let herself get into this predicament at all. It could probably have been avoided if she had checked the bus time-table.*

✔ *She also could have arranged for someone to accompany her, or, if possible, not to work after hours.*

✔ *She should have been aware of all the conditions regarding the bus stop's safety and risk factors.*

✔ *She described her "eerie" feeling as she walked down the office corridor, and relief to be out of the deserted building. Obviously she was anxious due to some intuitive feelings, and this should have told her to be on the alert. Also she was preoccupied about the dinner preparations while she was walking to the bus stop, and could not have been fully aware of what was going on around her.*

A DISABLED MAN AVOIDING STREET ASSAULT

I had just pulled a ligament while skiing, and the doctor said I could walk with a crutch or cane, whichever felt better, but not to overdo it. So when I went to work, I used the crutch and cane alternately and made the best of it.

Temporarily disabled people are at a greater disadvantage than people permanently disabled.

Being startled can immediately deprive you of valuable energy.

On the way home I had to pick up something at the cleaners, some distance from where I parked the car. On the way I noticed two boys walking towards me just about where the stores began. From their appearance and behavior I knew they were out for trouble. They were calling loud obscenities at me. One of them had a can of spray paint which he was using to mark up some of the buildings. Although I wanted to get out of this situation as fast as possible, I couldn't run, or even walk very fast.

I began *focusing* on everything around me, the number and location of parked cars, the amount of traffic, and the people nearby. Continuing to walk straight towards them would be a disaster, and there were no residential or office buildings for me to enter, just fences, a dead-end alley, and stores which had gone out of business. I did the relaxation and *imagery* exercises, hoping they would alleviate my fears and help me think more clearly.

Directly across the street was a parking lot, but I couldn't see an attendant from where I was, and didn't think any help would be available there. I was *feeling* frightened and desperate. There did not seem to be any way out. I kept up my survival exercises as long as I could. Then my eyes caught a large billboard, with one of those movable picture ads. I didn't notice the product, just that the guy was waving his arms, which gave me the idea.

I watched for more cars to drive by and made a fast, sharp left turn, maneuvering between two parked cars and out into the road. There was moderate traffic, and cars began blowing their horns all over the place. I thought, now is the time. I lifted up the cane and started waving it. I can't say why, it just seemed right at the time. No one knew what I was trying to do, but I sure created a hell of a lot of attention! And these two punks couldn't get at me. I saw them walk away down the street, no doubt looking for someone else and thinking that I was some loony. When they were well out of sight and I was sure I was out of harm's way, I made it back to my car, and drove home. On the way I waved over a police car and reported the whereabouts of these troublemakers.

Survival Skills Analysis

This is one of those situations with events occurring in too narrow a time frame to allow you to develop strategies easily. But his defensive survival psychology skills of *focusing* on what was happening on the street ahead of him, and *isolating* the approaching danger, enabled this man to prepare for action.

✔When he realized he had to make his move, he decisively followed his gut feelings, hoping that he would be successful. The holding mechanism was never permitted to operate.

A WOMAN FOLLOWED ONTO A BUS

Being so early it was not crowded as I entered the mall, and it was not until I had been to a few stores that I started to wonder if I was being followed. A tall, well-dressed man in his early forties always appeared to be not far from where I was.

As the stores started to fill up I felt better as it gave me some comfort to have more people around me. But still I had that gnawing feeling.

I decided to keep *focused,* and make sure I didn't reveal that I was on to him. I went on shopping in my usual way. It was difficult to be sure he was watching me, because he kept his distance.

When I spotted the cosmetic department I had an idea. I walked up to the cosmetician and asked for the free makeup consultation they were offering and sat down at the counter. When I adjusted the mirror there he was, staring right at me. The danger was clearly *isolated,* and I had a good view of him. His face was scarred, and his eyes deep set. He seemed very ill at ease. Up to now, he had been following me in motion, walking around as shoppers usually do. Now I was planted at this table, and this man didn't seem to know what to do.

As I was being made up, I kept him in view. He kept looking around as if he expected to be apprehended any moment. Suddenly, he disappeared from view, and my *feelings* changed to fright.

I had to compose myself. I went through the relaxation and *imagery* exercises, and started to think of my options. If I called a security guard and told him I suspected this man of following me, the guard would probably ask him for his ID. Then what? If I went to a public telephone booth to call the police, I was afraid I would be even more vulnerable. I discarded that idea too.

For most crimes, no arrests are ever made.

In the first seven to ten seconds of an attack, many victims describe their thought processes as confused, and filled with doubt that they would ever see their loved ones again.

I had to think of a way to safely get on and off the bus. I could not speak to the bus driver about my suspicions because I might be overheard, so that meant passing something written to him. The more I *imagined* what I would do the safer I felt. I was sure of my *technique* and that made me *feel* more confident.

I was prepared for him to follow me out of the store, so when I left I mingled with the crowds, staying close to at least one person. I knew he might follow me onto the bus, but as the bus stops at this time of day are usually crowded, I was pretty sure he wouldn't try anything there.

The bus arrived and several of us got on. I had hoped to get a seat near the driver, but there were none vacant. However, I was prepared. I gave the driver a five-dollar bill, and a note. He was annoyed, and said I had to have the right change. When he read the note he became quiet. It said: "Please have the police meet me at such and such street (which was not my address). A man in a brown plaid coat has been following me for two hours."

I sat as close to the driver as possible, and saw him watching the man very closely in his rearview mirror. I saw him pick up his microphone, and speak very softly. With the noise of the bus and other traffic no one on the bus could make out what he was saying.

We reached the place I had mentioned in the note, and I started to get off. Close behind was the man. I didn't see any police cars or, for that matter, anyone who looked like a cop. My heart sank. I wondered what had gone wrong, and why no one was there. But as soon as I stepped onto the curb, some men came out of nowhere. One grabbed my arm and gently moved me aside. The others grabbed the man, pinned his hands behind his back, and faced him against a wall. They searched him, and I saw them pull a mean-looking knife from his coat pocket.

The detective standing with me asked if I was all right. When I told him that I was, he asked me if I would come down to the police station and make out a statement.

Survival Skills Analysis

This woman certainly was *focused* and kept herself on top of the situation. Though at first she doubted her intuition, she never completely ignored it. She was able to *isolate* the danger signs, make good use of her environment, overcome her anxiety, evaluate her options appropriately, and choose a strategy.

✔*Her decision to board the bus was a correct one. Once on the bus, she knew she would be safe, since it is less likely that a criminal will attack someone in front of witnesses. She also knew that all buses have two-way radio communication systems.*

A WOMAN FOLLOWED WHILE JOGGING

I was anxious to run in my colorful and jazzy new sweatsuit. The weather was brisk and invigorating, and I got to the park early. I had been running about ten minutes when one of my shoes became untied. I stopped by a bench and as I leaned over to tie it I happened to glance back, and saw a man who must have been running behind me disappear into the bushes. There was no path where he went and I thought it odd. He wasn't dressed in the usual jogging garb. This didn't necessarily mean that he wasn't a jogger, but it made me suspicious.

By now the group I'd been running with was well ahead of me, and I was alone. I wasn't sure what to do. I couldn't catch up to them and thought of going back, but there was the chance this man might be waiting for me. I decided to continue running and stay alert, but I was worried that he might be waiting in the bushes for me. As I began to run I became more frightened. My intuition told me I was in danger. I stayed *focused* on everything around me, and tried to *isolate* anything that could mean danger.

Every so often I turned, and sure enough, could see him way behind me. He had on a sweater, jeans, and a knitted pull-over hat. As soon as he saw me turn around to look, he ducked into the bushes. He was definitely not a jogger, but maybe I couldn't outrun him anyway. I knew I had to outsmart him. I tried to become more aware of my *feelings*. I was scared, but relieved to know where he was. I had been jogging here so long I knew every curve in the road. I hoped he did not. There was a turn coming up where I knew I would be out of his view for a few minutes. I thought that I could use this to my advantage but wasn't sure

The divorced, separated, or never married rather than the married or widowed are in general more likely to be victims of crime.

*The situation always
dictates the
response.*

how. I had to decide upon a *technique.* I couldn't confront him, and hiding was out as my new jogging suit would serve as a beacon for him. The only feasible way out was running.

I was pretty sure that if I cut through the wooded area I would reach the trail again and find the group.

When the blind curve was between us, I made a sharp turn into the underbrush, and kept on going as fast as I could without looking back. It seemed like I was traveling forever. I was becoming winded and tired, mostly from fright. But I felt I couldn't stop. I'd made my decision that this was how I was going to escape.

I began my breathing and *imagery* exercises which certainly helped me keep up my endurance. I was coming to what looked like a clearing. It was the trail! I felt a new vigor, but as I reached it, I found it was deserted. I was so sure I'd caught up with the group. I wondered if I could have misjudged the distance. I stood for a few moments to catch my breath and gather my wits, and then I heard them. I'd come out ahead of them. I couldn't believe it. As they reached me, I began waving my hands so they would stop. I told my story, and we all proceeded out of the park together to look for a police officer. We found one, and I gave him the man's description.

Survival Skills Analysis

The woman in this situation had limited options. There was a chance that she couldn't outrun her follower, and she was alone. In view of these circumstances, her strategy was correct: she *focused* on what was happening, *isolated* the danger signs, and paid proper attention to her intuition.

A WOMAN ASSAULTED IN AN ELEVATOR

I decided to go straight home from work rather than stop off at the store for a few items. As I walked into my apartment building, everything looked normal. I wasn't being followed and the lobby looked clear. As the elevator arrived, I heard the lock on the outside door buzz, and saw the lobby door swing open. I stepped into the elevator and the door was beginning to close when this man came darting across the lobby, directly towards me. My first inclination was to run past him out the elevator while the door was still open. But in that split second of my hesitation he was inside, and it was too late. I wanted to believe that this was just someone who was in a big hurry and meant no harm, but my intuition told me differently. He was dirty-looking, shabbily dressed in stained clothing. His face was unshaven. He wasn't very young, about forty, I thought.

As the door closed, he lunged at me. I was so scared, I backed up into the front corner next to the control panel. This was a good move since he could not get behind me, and I gained some leverage by bracing myself against the wall. I had no intention of letting him rape me.

I was *feeling* terrorized, vulnerable, and angry. But I think that my anger outweighed everything else.

"Take off your clothes," he said.

I didn't move. He grabbed my blouse and tried to open it, and I resisted. As we struggled, I managed to press most of the buttons on the control panel.

By this time, the elevator was approaching the third floor. My apartment was on the sixth floor. We stopped on the third and the door opened, but no one was there. I struggled to get out, but it was no use. The door closed.

Now he was getting angrier, and his hands went for the STOP button. I would not let him get to it. He could not keep me under control and at the same time control the elevator. I began screaming as loud as I could, and I could see this unnerved him. We were approaching the fourth floor. He hadn't revealed any weapon, but I didn't know how I was going to get out of this.

When the door opened on the fourth floor, he held on to me tighter, at the same time trying to get my clothes off. I began screaming again, hoping I would be heard, and as we struggled, I managed to hit the ALARM button. It went off, but in order for it to go on sounding, I had to hold it down. He got angrier and began slapping me.

I ignored this, and convinced myself that since he had no weapon I was going to defend myself at all costs.

At floor number five the door opened, and again there was no one. He was making some headway undressing me, but I was still resisting and screaming.

The violent crime rates of the 1960s and 1970s coincided with the baby-boom generation coming of age.

1990 was the beginning of a new crime-wave.

On our way to the sixth and top floor I thought of the stairs to the roof. That really frightened me. He was becoming more and more forceful. I continued screaming.

I thought that if he intended to rape me on the roof I might have more of a chance to escape, but I also thought of the risk of being thrown from the roof. I tried some breathing and imagery exercises, but wasn't sure how much they helped.

The panel light showed we were at the sixth floor. As the door opened, I decided to go limp. I lay motionless on the floor of the elevator, hearing him cursing at me, calling me obscenities. Any moment I expected to be dragged to the roof, raped, or killed. Still cursing, he started to kick me—hard. I knew I must not move. He was hurting me badly. I said to myself, "I have to endure this. It's better than being raped, or killed." As he continued kicking, I blocked out his cursing, and repeated this phrase to myself over and over. I thought it would never end, but I remained perfectly still. All of a sudden he stopped. I heard the door close, and nothing more. The car started to move down. Then it stopped, and opened again. I heard talking and opened my eyes. I saw a man and woman waiting to get on. I was still slumped on the floor where I'd fallen.

Slowly I stood up. I told them what had happened, and they accompanied me to my apartment. I immediately called the police, and described my assailant and the assault.

When they arrived, I mentioned all the precautions I had taken, and could not understand how this could have happened to me. They explained that many assailants wait in hiding for someone to go into a building, and then press all the apartment buttons. Usually someone will open the door without checking the person's identity, and they rely on this.

Survival Skills Analysis

Though this woman had *focused* correctly on her surroundings, she could not have been prepared for this situation, or anticipated it.

✔*Her initial intuitive feelings to run out of the elevator were correct. This would, of course, have broken the holding mechanism. (Though there is always the chance that her assailant would have run after her. Things happen so fast in an assault situation, one cannot always behave rapidly enough.)*

✔*Once in the assault situation, she did all she could to survive. When she became aware of what her attacker was going to do, she placed herself (unintentionally at first) in a more advantageous place near the control panel.*

✔*She also did other correct things: pressing all the floor stops on the panel, trying to prevent her assailant from stopping the elevator, and screaming to attract attention.*

✔*When everything else failed, her decision to place herself in a physically disabled state proved effective.*

A WOMAN BEING FOLLOWED

I'd already run errands at the post office and the library. I was now leaving the dentist's and debating whether to walk the long or the short way to meet my friend. The long way would be populated, and there were stores, while the short way consisted of just office and residential buildings. Since I was late, I decided on the short way.

I was waiting at a corner for the traffic light to change when I noticed him—an ordinary-looking middle-aged man, with grayish thinning hair, wearing slacks and a short leather jacket. Suddenly, things started to click into place. I remembered seeing him earlier in one of the lines at the post office. Also in the library I had seen him wandering around while I was waiting at the counter. And now he was across the street, about a block behind me. I found it hard to believe that this was a coincidence. But as it was equally hard to believe that he was stalking me I started to doubt my intuition.

I had to calm down to see just how scared I was *feeling*, and how I could get myself out of this. I was safe enough for the moment so I started my relaxation and *imagery* exercises and began to *feel* more in control. I desperately wanted to keep him in view, because as long as I knew where he was, there could be no surprises. Without any idea of my

Hearing harsh and violent dictates from an assailant diminishes victims' self-esteem, and gives them the impression they have no choice but to listen.

next move, I continued walking. I tried to find out where he was by making believe I had something in my shoe and leaning against a lamp pole to empty it. I saw he had crossed to my side.

When I reached the next corner the light was in my favor, and I crossed to the other side. I wondered if he would follow me. I had a difficult time keeping myself from turning around, and this cat-and-mouse game was wearing me down. Just then, a truck carrying huge sheets of glass along its sides turned the corner. In the reflection I saw he was right behind me. There was now no question that I was being stalked.

He was still maintaining his distance, but I feared this would not last much longer. All this time, I had been looking for some way to get help: a cab, a police car, a policeman, a truck stopping for a delivery, any way to attract attention, but there was none. I thought of running into an apartment house or office building, but was afraid of being trapped in the hallway or elevator before I could get to someone. I decided to stay out in the open where my chances were better, but my fear was beginning to increase and it looked like there was no way out.

About a block and a half ahead, a taxi was pulling over to let out a couple. I turned around and noticed the man walking faster. It had to be now, I thought. I started to run towards the cab, waving my arms screaming, "Help! Police! Fire!" The woman stopped and looked towards me. I kept on screaming and waving my arms, but I couldn't go on. Totally out of breath, I collapsed on the pavement. Though I was conscious I couldn't get up. The couple ran over to me, but before I could say anything, the man also reached me.

He said to them, "It's OK. She's a friend of mine. I'll take care of her."

I grabbed the sleeve of the woman tightly and panted, "Don't believe him. He's been following me for hours. Call the police."

By now, the driver, a huge man who looked like a wrestler, was out of the car, and had heard me. The cabbie asked him for ID and he turned and ran. Though we knew he couldn't be charged with anything the driver called the police from his cab and we filed a report.

Survival Skills Analysis

If this woman had *focused* more on the people around during her errands, she might have noticed the man and become suspicious earlier, and not have taken the shorter, less-populated route.

> Most people, after they have been stripped of their valuables, have a feeling of helplessness.

✔She did remember seeing her would-be assailant in the post office and library, thus isolating the possible danger.

✔She did use her intuition before it became too late, when she started to question the afternoon's coincidences.

Stalking has been clearly identified as one of the serious crime categories, and the emotional aftermath to its victims can be devastating. The stalker, like the rapist, has deep unmet psychological needs which make themselves known in pathologically dangerous behavior, and as with a rapist, trying to reason with him is useless.

A CAR DRIVER ATTACKED BY A GANG OF YOUTHS

As I was having mechanical trouble with my car, I decided to take the short route home from my meeting. I hoped the directions I'd been given were right because I hadn't been in the area before. As I drove, I couldn't see the names of the streets in the directions, and the neighborhood was getting worse and worse. (My husband had suggested I take the portable CB along in case I got lost, but I'd assured him that wouldn't happen.) It was then the engine began making a strange noise. It finally slowed to a stop and stalled. I tried repeatedly to start it, but it was no use. I didn't want to wear the battery down, so I let it be.

I knew I had to attract someone's attention to get help. I quickly got out of the car, opened the hood, got back in, and locked all the doors. I thought of putting on my bright lights or my emergency flashers. But since I couldn't start the engine, and didn't want to wear the battery down, I decided to wait. As I looked around, I had a feeling of danger lurking. The area was deserted, dusk was approaching, and I was getting scared. I thought of going out and looking for someone, but then I was afraid of who I might find, so I decided against it.

My intuition wasn't wrong. Leaning against a fence down the road were three youths who looked like gang members. They were wearing black jackets with colored emblems and writing which I couldn't make out, and were looking hard in my direction. I had visions of something terrible about to happen to me. They weren't moving, except for some clubs they were swinging.

"This couldn't possibly be happening to me" is a dangerous pattern of thought.

Before long, they began to stroll towards me. Difficult as it was, I began my relaxation and *imagery* exercises. They reached the car. Just their appearance sent shivers through me. Two of them walked around the car while one was looking inside at me and grinning. He motioned to me with his hand to open the window. I rolled it down less than an inch.

"Whatsa matter lady, you stuck?" he asked me in a low drawl, while chewing gum, and I nodded my head. He said, "That's too bad, ain't it fellas?" and they all said in chorus. "Sure is."

I knew this taunting game was the prelude to trouble. Then he said, "Maybe we can help. Think we can help fellas?" They all answered again in chorus, "Maybe."

"He said, "Got any money? We all can't do much without money, can we fellas?"

I *focused* on the street ahead, which was still deserted. A few low broken-down apartment buildings were on my right. On the left were some stores which were closed, and farther down was an open vacant lot. I looked in my rearview mirror but didn't see anything different. My hopes for getting out of this ordeal were fading, but I'd noticed a cross street about two city blocks ahead of me with some traffic. My only hope was to attract somebody there. Meanwhile I had to keep my eyes on what my assailants were doing.

I was thinking of a plan, and was *imagining* the *technique* I would use, wondering if it would work, at the same time trying to calm myself, and continue my *imagery* exercises..

Then one of them said, "Well, where's the money?"

I opened my purse, took out all the bills I had and passed them through the opening in the window.

He grabbed the bills, counted them, and said, "That's all? You won't make us happy with just that, will she fellas?" Again, they all shook their heads and said, "No." Then their leader said, "Well, then, I guess it's show time, ain't it fellas?" They began slowly rocking the car. I was becoming sick to my stomach, but had to keep my eyes on the cross street ahead. I was debating whether I should wait until I saw some traffic or just go ahead with my plan. They were rocking the car harder and faster. One shut the hood, and began to climb up on it. I knew I couldn't wait any longer and leaned on the horn. He jumped about five feet and looked really angry. I kept on with the horn, and began flashing my low and high beams.

One was trying to break the window and get at me. One was trying to open the hood, which couldn't be unlocked from the outside. Frustrated, he began smashing in the hood. The third attacker was at my right door trying to smash the window. They were making headway, and I was still sounding the horn and flashing my lights.

My window was nearly smashed through when I heard sirens and saw flashing lights. Two police cars from opposite directions converged on us. The thugs had nowhere to run, and were quickly put up against a wall, disarmed, searched, handcuffed, and put in the back of one of the police cars.

A trucker had seen the flashing lights and heard the horn. He didn't know what was wrong but thought it should be checked out so he called the precinct.

Survival Skills Analysis

✔Using a car which is not mechanically sound to go to an unfamiliar place is definitely a bad idea.

✔Using directions without first checking the route and destination on a map was also poor judgment.

✔By the time this woman focused on the area, believed her intuition, and isolated the danger she was in, it was already too late. But considering the circumstances, she did the only thing she could, which was to stay in the car even though the risk factors were many. Outside there were more, and she would have had no protection whatsoever. Nor would she have been able to use the car as she did to attract attention.

✔She was wise to conserve the battery until she absolutely needed it.

A MIDDLE-OF-THE-NIGHT BREAK-IN

It was about 2:00 a.m. when I heard a noise downstairs. I knew it wasn't a dream or my imagination. I waited a few seconds, and then I heard it again.

I was scared and I didn't know what to do. It sounded as if someone

Victims of household crimes, such as burglary, are more likely to be renters than homeowners.

Blacks, rather than whites or other minority groups, are more likely to be victims of violent crime.

was in the house. I knew if I woke my husband he would want to go downstairs to investigate. But if I did nothing, and the intruder came upstairs and awakened him, anything could happen. So I nudged him gently. As he lifted his head off the pillow, I put my hand over his mouth whispering, "Sh-h, someone's downstairs."

Just at that moment, there was more noise. It was unmistakable. He sat up and looked as if he was about to get out of bed. I grabbed his arm. "All the books I've read say that when something like this happens, make believe you're sleeping," I said. "All a robber wants is to steal, and not have to confront or hurt anyone."

But he whispered, "You got it a little wrong, honey. You only should make believe you're sleeping if you are awakened and find a robber in your room. In a situation like this we should try to get out of the house or call the cops.

I said, "How can we get out? There's no way we can get downstairs without making noise, and we certainly can't climb out the window."

"OK" Marty said, as he picked up the phone receiver, and ducked under the blankets. I started using my relaxation and *imagery* exercises. I know they helped get me through this ordeal.

Marty put the phone back, and soon we heard our intruder come up the stairs. At that point, we both turned over and made believe we were asleep. My heart felt as if it was going to pop out of my body, but I continued my relaxation exercises as best I could. He started going through the drawers, and we heard our belongings being tossed from side to side. If you never had this happen to you, you can't imagine the feelings: the intrusion, the fright, not knowing what might happen next. After a few moments, he left. We heard the front door close and everything was quiet again.

A few minutes passed, and we still didn't hear anything. We got out of bed and looked around. The drawers to our dresser and bureau and night tables were open. Everything inside was moved around. But nothing else was disturbed. We were lucky.

Survival Skills Analysis

The things this woman and her husband had read may have saved both their lives. Being able to convince the robber that they were truly asleep and represented no risk to him was the key to their survival.

Housebreakers rarely welcome a confrontation. Whenever possible, they prefer to get in and out of the house as quickly as possible.

If this robber had provoked a confrontation (highly unlikely since they were both committed to feigning sleep), this could have led to violence.

COMING UPON AN APARTMENT ROBBER

My neighbor was away, and I had agreed to water her plants and check to see if everything in the apartment was all right. With all the crime going on, we'd decided to do this for each other a few years ago. Since she was due back in two days, I thought I would stop on the way home from the library for a few food items for her. I bought more than I'd intended, and was annoyed at myself for having to carry such a heavy bundle of groceries plus my library books.

As I didn't feel like bending to put the packages down, I held onto them while I opened the door. When I put the key in the lock it didn't turn as it usually does. But I was certain I had locked the door after I left a few days ago. I tried the knob and it turned easily—too easily. For a second, I hesitated about entering, but then went in anyway.

As soon as I opened the door, I saw a man standing no more than twenty feet from me. We were equally startled. He began to run towards me. I had no idea whether he was going to attack me or run past me out the door.

I *thought* fast and, holding my packages and books like a basketball, threw them with all my might directly at his head. It caught him off guard long enough for me to turn and run down the stairs to the lobby. Once outside, I screamed for help. The man quickly followed me out of the building, but ran in the opposite direction.

I called the police from another neighbor's home and gave them a description of the robber. I also asked them to send someone over to re-cylinder the lock.

Survival Skills Analysis

✔The moment this woman saw that the lock wasn't working correctly, and the doorknob turned easily, she should have dropped her bundles and run down the stairs. If the elevator was still on her floor, she should have taken it.

No matter how unprovoked, most victims of violence feel a certain amount of guilt about what has happened to them.

> Household crimes can leave victims feeling devastated and unsafe.

✔She admitted not paying attention to her intuition when she was hesitant about entering the apartment.

✔When she entered the apartment she did exactly the right thing by trying to get away from the intruder as fast as possible.

✔Her escape was successful because of her ability to think and act decisively.

✔She succeeded by using the techniques of surprise and distraction when she threw her bundles at him to gain a little time. Doing so broke the holding mechanism.

USING CLUES TO AVOID VIOLENT CONFRONTATION

It was awful weather, pouring rain, and I was glad my friend was giving me a ride home that day. When we came to my house, she pulled into the driveway to let me out and then drove away. I unlocked and opened the front door, and noticed the carpet was wet. Since everyone had been out all day, I was suspicious. I glanced round, and *focused* on the den.

The den is directly ahead as you come in. It's always untidy because it's used for sewing and ironing, and we always keep the door closed, even when we go out. The door was open.

At that point, I felt someone had been, or still was, in the house. I knew I had to do something fast. I backed out the door, closed it to lock as quietly as I could, ran across the street to my neighbor, and called the police.

Several police cars arrived quietly without their sirens. The officers met me at my neighbor's house, and I gave one of them my house key. Several officers entered the house while the others surrounded it. Soon after they came out with someone in handcuffs.

Survival Skills Analysis

This young woman used everything she had learned from defensive-survival psychology. She immediately *focused* on her surroundings, *isolated* the possible danger signs, followed her intuition, and acted decisively.

A VICTIM OF A STREET ASSAULT

It was later than usual when I left work, and I was surprised to find the street deserted. It unnerved me a bit. I thought of going back to the building and waiting for someone to walk me to the subway, but was too embarrassed to ask. So I tried to concentrate on something pleasant—a surprise birthday party I was planning for a friend.

All I remember next was a strong arm grabbing me around the neck from behind, a hand tightly over my mouth, and a gruff voice saying, "Be quiet or I'll kill you!"

It's amazing how fast fear and panic can totally paralyze you. Thoughts of rape, robbery, and murder all went racing through my mind.

I was too immobilized physically and psychologically to try and pull his hand away or scream. As he was dragging me to what looked like some kind of alley, I became nauseous, and felt my legs go limp. I'm getting sick, I thought. That gave me an idea of a technique I could use. I clutched my chest and said just loudly enough for him to hear, "My heart." Then I just let myself drop.

For a moment I heard nothing. I decided to stay quiet and play dead. Eventually I felt my purse being pulled from my shoulder, and then heard footsteps going away and disappearing. Very slowly I opened my eyes. There were no signs of him. I got up, but was still so weak I was barely able to stand. I made my way back to the street by clinging on to the buildings. A motorist finally stopped, and I told him what had happened. He took me back to where I work and we called the police..

Survival Skills Analysis

When this woman left her building she was not *focused*, she did not *isolate* any sources of danger, nor did she pay attention to her intuition. She could not have done much more that was wrong.

✔ *She should have followed her first inclination to have someone accompany her.*

✔ *Her decision to concentrate on something pleasant prevented her from concentrating on her surroundings.*

Households headed by younger people are more susceptible to break-ins and robberies.

✔In addition, it is quite possible that the anxiety she was feeling on find-ing the street deserted was reflected in her body language—something assailants are astute at assessing.

✔When she fell down, her body became totally dead-weight, which made it more difficult for her attacker to handle her. If his intentions were to rape her, he would have had to move her body by himself in order to complete the sex act. If he had wanted to harm her, it now looked like she was already harmed (her heart). If he only intended to rob her, he accomplished his goal.

> The psychology of mob violence stretches the boundaries of acceptable behavior.

A STREET ATTACK BY A GANG

My wife and I had been to a concert. I suggested that we top off the eve-ning with a snack, and walk to a restaurant in the vicinity. My wife was reluctant because the neighborhood was fairly deserted and the hour was late, but I convinced her the walk would do us good.

We had not gone far when we turned a corner and saw four youths approaching us. They were dressed in boots, torn jeans, leather and denim jackets, and caps and bandannas. My wife was clearly scared.

I told her to watch me closely in case I got an idea, and be ready to follow my lead quickly.

They became louder and more boisterous as they got closer. Two moved out into the road while the other two moved closer to the build-ing, forcing us to walk between them. The two closest on either side stretched their arms over our heads to form a bridge as they passed us. But then they stopped demanding our money and jewelry.

I took out my wallet, and started to take off my watch and ring. My wife did the same and they shoved everything into their pockets.

I had hoped this would be the end of it, but they then turned their attention to my wife. Almost automatically I had begun to do the relax-ation and *imagery* exercises. In my gut I knew the worst was to come, and I feared for both of us.

"Say now, you wouldn't mind if we kind of all shared her—just for tonight you understand—would you?"

At this point, no one had shown any kind of weapon, but there was no way that we could enter into a physical confrontation. I scanned the area, desperately looking for something. About three-quarters of a block away I saw some men loading newspapers into a truck. In some way I knew I had to distract our assailants and attract the truckers.

I quickly *imagined* the *technique*, with my words and actions, and how I was going to alert my wife about it. I had been holding her hand and now started to alternately squeeze it, and palpate her palm with my fingers, hoping she'd know that I was giving her a signal to watch me and be ready to act.

I looked up to the sky, pointed, and screamed at the top of my lungs "Look out!"

Everyone, including my wife, looked skyward. I tightened my grip on my wife's hand and started running into the road, pulling her with me, yelling "Run, run!"

I headed diagonally across the road and down the block towards the truckers.

"Help!" we yelled. "We've just been robbed!"

Our assailants ran after us, but when they saw the truckers drop their bundles they retreated. The truckers caught them and called the police, who got there quickly.

Survival Skills Analysis

Isolated areas and late hours are prime conditions for assailants. Had the proper precautions been taken this couple's evening would not have ended in near disaster. Once they met their attackers it was too late to escape.

This man used his survival skills to their maximum, as well as his creativity.

A WOMAN ATTACKED IN AN APARTMENT-HOUSE STAIRWAY

I was bringing my mother a small cellular telephone so she could always reach someone, even when she went out.

On the elevator door a sign read, "Elevator Out of Order," and I had to walk up six flights. The stairs were not well lighted, and intuition told me

The increasing number of murders is not limited to one geographical area, or to any social or economic category.

Law enforcement and community programs are finding it increasingly difficult to provide the protection the public expects.

to turn around and leave. But since I was already there, I thought I might as well go on. It was important that my mother have this new phone.

Halfway up the second flight of stairs, a man appeared behind me. I was frightened, and almost automatically began using the relaxation and *imagery* exercises. He was on the first flight and maintaining the distance between us. I started to wonder if I could be wrong about my feelings of danger, and was overreacting.

I was now approaching the fourth flight. I knew he was at least a flight behind but didn't want to look. Approaching the fifth flight, I knew I had to get a grip on myself. I knew what I was *feeling:* my heart was pounding, my legs were shaking, and my mind was full of fear. I had to prepare myself emotionally for immediate action at even the slightest opportunity. I tried to think of solutions like turning around, running at him and knocking him down. Suddenly one flight above me appeared another man. He was at least in his forties, had dark hair, and was wearing a sweater and jeans. He just stood there looking at me.

I now felt that there was no possible way to escape harm. No matter how hard I *focused,* I could not come up with any choices. There were only blank plaster walls, steel railings, concrete steps, and an isolated and soundproofed area all around me. But at that instant, my eyes caught a sign on the wall directly behind him: "Say No to Drugs!" I thought quickly and shouted in an authoritative way, "Get the hell out of here! You're in the middle of a drug bust! This place will be swarming with police within minutes!" I opened my purse, pulled out the phone and started to talk into it. "Units one and two, hold off for a minute. I got two guys up here who could really foul things up."

The man above came racing down the stairs, nearly knocking me over, and the one below disappeared. I went up to my mother's apartment and called the police from there. When they arrived I gave them a description of the two, so that they could put out a bulletin.

Survival Skills Analysis

This woman's life needn't have been in jeopardy if she had simply said yes to her intuition, as she almost did.

✔*In a situation like this, when someone entering a building is being set up, no amount of focusing would help. Assailants lying in wait always have an advantage. This is why she should have isolated the potential danger immediately when she saw the sign on the elevator.*

✔*Her technique and the way she carried it out were effective in breaking the holding mechanism, but, of course, avoiding the situation would have been far safer.*

A WOMAN AVOIDING ASSAULT ON A DESERTED STREET

I drove downtown to my doctor's and was glad to find a parking space even though it was a few blocks away on a side street.

As I was returning to the car after my appointment, the street looked deserted, except for a man reading a newspaper leaning against a building across from my car. He had a beard, and was not especially clean looking. I was reluctant to approach my car, and my intuition told me that this could be dangerous. I started to slow up but didn't want to make it obvious that I was suspicious. I was afraid to turn and run for fear he might run after me. I wondered if he had an accomplice that I couldn't see. This thought brought out all kinds of *feelings*—fright, worry, anger, vulnerability.

I began doing my relaxation and *imagery* exercises as I walked. A huge moving van began to turn the corner and was almost parallel with me. I thought for a moment and saw my chance to retreat without my would-be assailant seeing me. By the time the van passed, I was around the corner in the midst of people. I wondered how I would ever get to my car safely.

I decided to wait for a police car and hail it. But when I finally saw a patrol car approaching, it was on the wrong side of the road, and the officer didn't see me. Time was passing and I really had to get back home.

I stood in the street wondering what to do. I thought of going back to the doctor's office and having the nurse call police headquarters. But that would make me very late getting home. I thought of going into a store and telling the storekeeper, or stopping a stranger and having him walk with me to the car. As I stood pondering these things, a taxi

Assault invariably shakes a victim's self-esteem, leaving them feeling more vulnerable than before.

> *Wear your jewelry out of sight: necklaces inside your shirt; bracelets to the inside of your sleeve; gems on rings turned to the inside of the palm.*

stopped to let a passenger out. I thought fast and, without hesitating, hopped in the back and told the driver my plight.

He drove around the block, and I pointed out where the car was parked. The man was still there. The taxi driver pulled up next to my car and waited until I started the engine.

I pulled out of the space and proceeded slowly towards the corner, watching the man in my rear-view mirror. From out of who knows where, I saw another man walk over to him. They were both looking in my direction. As I reached the next corner, I saw a police car. I waved it over, told the officers what had happened, and gave them a complete description of the two men.

Survival Skills Analysis

This woman *focused* on the right things, *isolated* the danger, and paid attention to her intuition. She was also able to act decisively, making a split-second decision to get into the taxi. This was probably the best of all the options she had available. Taking the taxi insured her safety and did not allow the holding mechanism to come into play.

A WOMAN STOPPED ON THE STREET

It was a beautiful day. I almost wished it was stormy so that I wouldn't feel I was missing much by having to spend it indoors at this very posh fund-raiser my friend and I were attending. I also did not particularly like having to dress up and put on expensive jewelry, but I felt I had to fit in.

As we headed home, away from the mansions and limousines, and nearer to our neighborhood, I asked my friend to drop me off, so that I could walk the rest of the way and take advantage of the weather.

I was already halfway home, when I remembered that I was supposed to pick up some manuscripts for my husband. I was going to do this on the way home with my friend because the neighborhood wasn't good, and she could wait for me. I was only a few blocks away. I hesitated, but decided to go anyway. As I approached my destination, the streets became noticeably more deserted, and that made me uneasy. I was about to turn around and go back when I noticed a landmark that my husband had told me was near the building I was seeking, so I continued. I was concentrating on looking for the number of the building, and did not see the man who was heading in my direction until he was practically upon me.

He stopped directly in front of me, causing me to pause. Politely he asked a question, but as he spoke, he was looking at my jewelry, sparkling in the sun.

I felt suspicious and afraid. My intuition told me to be careful, and not to stop or answer him. I thought for a second, sidestepped, quickened my pace, and headed across the street in the direction of a delivery truck that had just parked. As I began crossing, I heard him say loudly, "Hey, I just wanted to..." and then his voice trailed off. I was certain that this was no accidental meeting, and that I was being set up. I didn't look back, but was pretty sure that he had decided not to pursue me. As I reached the driver of the truck he was about to do some unloading.

I told him what had happened and he said he'd take me home. It was less than a mile to my house, but I decided not to give him the address and had him drop me at a corner nearby.

I thanked the driver, hung around until I was sure he was well out of sight, and made my way to my friend's house first, just as a precaution, and waited there for my husband to pick me up on his way home.

Survival Skills Analysis

Once again, this woman got herself into a situation that never had to happen, by doing all the wrong things.

✔ *First, she should have let her friend take her straight home, and not tried to pick up her husband's manuscript dressed as she was in a bad neighborhood. Having her friend waiting for her would have done little good if she was attacked in the building.*

✔ *Her initial intuition told her not to go on the errand. She disregarded it. Her intuition to turn around when the area was deserted was also ignored.*

✔ *Then she was so preoccupied with locating the building number, she was not focused on her surroundings, and was therefore unable to isolate the danger signs, never seeing the threat until faced with it.*

Anger safely expressed is preferable to anger festering inside.

Keep only one eye on an altercation or "problem" in the street. It could be a diversion or trap.

✔Fortunately she had her wits about her from here on, and behaved correctly. By not stopping, and instead speeding up, and crossing the street, she actually broke the holding mechanism, not allowing herself to become identified as a victim, and not giving her would-be assailant time to implement his plan of action.

Epilogue

I HOPE THIS BOOK will cause you to take some serious steps towards your own self-preservation. Once you learn to use your mind/body connection, it can help you to:

✔ *Change certain attitudes and behavior to decrease your susceptibility to physical assault.*

✔ *Activate your inner warning system in the face of danger before it is too late.*

✔ *Avoid panic, rationally evaluate your options, and defend yourself by acting appropriately.*

Victimization can happen to you. A survival attitude is absolutely necessary, and with it you can create an edge for yourself when faced with assault. You can control threatening events, rather than allowing them to control you.

Fear and panic are normal, appropriate, and permissible. Stifling them is not your objective, nor is it realistic to do so. But being able to control your fear and behaving in a more productive way are your objectives. Practicing relaxation and imagery skills will help you minimize some of the automatic panic reactions that arise in a dangerous situation, and will also help you act more productively. Without having established a personal training regimen, being able to react effectively and on cue in a panic situation is unlikely for most people. Practice and rehearse all you have learned and imagine your own scenarios for survival.

No book can guarantee that you are going to survive a life-threatening situation, nor can it answer all your questions. Throughout this book, I have continually stressed the importance of creativity for survival. No matter how many or how few of this book's suggestions you carry away with you, this one should top the list.

But assailants can be as creative as their most creative victim. They can impersonate priests, beggars, delivery men, repair men, even law enforcement officers. They will engage in some of the most outlandish trickery to distract you and keep you off guard in order to gain entry into your car, your office, or your home. Keep the holding mechanism in mind, and always be wary of anyone, doing or saying anything to cause you to stop what you are doing. Whether you are walking, jogging, bicycling, or driving your car; whether at work, school, or play THINK SURVIVAL.

The survival techniques described in this book can teach you how to develop your own physical power and psychological strength. They are the only sensible weapons a civilized society can offer in an uncivilized world of violence.

APPENDIX I

How to Describe an Assailant

When you have survived an assault, knowing how to describe your attacker will be vital, and your awareness skills will play a dominant role. The elements of a good description are sex, race, approximate age, height and weight ranges.

BUILD: *Fat, thin, muscular, stocky.*

COMPLEXION: *Light, medium, albino, dark, ruddy, olive, yellow.*

HAIR: *Color, length. Whether crew cut, thick, curly, receding, wavy, bushy, thinning, kinky, Afro, wig, bald.*

FACE: *Thin, long, broad, angular, round, oval, high cheek bones.*

FACIAL HAIR: *Amount. Mustache, goatee, beard, unshaven, sideburns.*

FACIAL ODDITIES: *Birthmarks, acne, acne scars, pockmarks, moles, freckles.*

FACIAL SCARS: *Nose, cheeks, lips, forehead, eyebrows.*

EYES: *Color, size. Whether crossed, squinting, bulging.*

EYEBROWS: *Color. Whether thin, heavy, bushy, medium.*

EARS: *Size. Close to head, protruding, pierced, cauliflower, deformed.*

NOSE: *Size. Crooked, straight, hooked, upturned, broad, thin, fat. Large, small nostrils.*

CHIN: *Long, pointed, square, protruding.*

LIPS: *Thin, thick, wide, small.*

TEETH: *Healthy, broken, missing, false, decayed, stained, protruding, irregular.*

BODY SCARS: *On arms, hands, wrist, neck, chest, head, legs, feet.*

MISCELLANEOUS: *Noticeable birthmarks, tattoos, deformities, clothes, jewelry, habits, mannerisms.*

APPENDIX II:

Selecting a Self-Defense Program

Survival must be a combination of proactive and reactive behavior. Proactive methods have been discussed in this book. Reactive methods, such as those taught in martial arts school, should consist of updated realistic techniques, proven to be effective in uncontrollable situations. Remember, the type of weaponry on the streets today did not exist centuries ago, when the martial arts were established.

Selecting a self-defense program is very personal, and each fills diverse psychological and physical needs which will differ from person to person. In this quest, there are some important factors to consider:

✔ *Validate the instructor's qualifications. Qualifications can be exaggerated. All titles and certificates should state the methodology used to attain credentials, and the dates awarded, so you can know the length of time the person has been instructing. I recommend that anyone teaching self-defense have a minimum of ten years experience in the field of self-protection.*

✔ *Check into the instructional history. Find out how long the school has been in existence, and the reputation of the instructor giving the courses. Seek out past students. See how they liked the program, and how much they remembered.*

✔ *Make sure the instructor is seasoned. Teaching the hands-on reality of defending yourself must come from a person who knows the streets. A seasoned instructor will have first-hand knowledge, and the experience of being in altercations. Those with backgrounds in security and law-enforcement enhance their instructional abilities.*

✔ *Beware of the financial hype. While you can learn much in eight weeks when the focus is properly placed, do not believe the gimmick which says you will become a lethal weapon at the end of this time. This is nothing more than an ego boost to make you feel you are something you are not. No one can learn proper weapon disarming techniques, or defense against multiple attackers in so short a time.*

✔ *Good instructors will train their students to read potentially dangerous situations and how to avoid them at all costs. Instruction should be designed to focus on basic techniques catered to one's ability, size, and strength, and should build confidence, not egos.*

APPENDIX III:
FOR PSYCHOLOGISTS AND INTERESTED OTHERS

A Defensive Survival Psychology Group Program —escape from abuse

This program is both preventive and therapeutic in nature, being based upon the principles described in the preceding chapters. It deals with [1] ways that people disallow or inhibit their body from physically expressing itself [2] their lack of physical spontaneity in life-threatening situations [3] how they behave on a nonverbal level in the context of interpersonal relationships where one must physically respond to others [4] how all this translates into interpretive action states.

The program is group rather than individually oriented because this approach is the most effective and expeditious way to achieve our goals, and the mix of participants is important towards this end. The cooperative interaction and reinforcement occurring between and among the participants, groups and leaders is what makes the program effective and produces optimal results. The process is known as synergism. The more heterogeneous, the more productive the sessions will be. Therefore, individuals are encouraged to join who may have experienced victimization directly (first hand), indirectly (been witness to it), concerned about their own safety, or just interested in preventive measures that can be applied in a violent society. It is also for professional therapists who want to learn more about this whole approach to the prevention and treatment of abuse and victimization.

The essential elements involve a combination of physical and psychological techniques, utilizing such things as relaxation procedures, guided imagery, enactment of actual crime scenarios, and role playing.

For more information about the Defensive Survival Psychology Program or to order tapes of the relaxation and imagery scripts please write:

The New Jersey Network for Crime Victim Protection Inc.
PO Box 120
Paramus, New Jersey
07653-0120

ACKNOWLEDGEMENTS

I want to especially acknowledge Thomas Patire, who served as my technical advisor, and provided the expertise related to the physical and environmental aspects of prevention and survival, as well as scenarios from his own experience, presented in the chapter entitled "Survival Techniques in Action."

The talents of Michael DePasquale Jr. and Vincent Marchetti helped to make the chapter titled "Tips and Techniques for the Disabled and Elderly" meaningful to a group of special people.

I am grateful to Richard Diamond, Michael Held, and Warren Williams for sharing some personal aspects of their lives.

A valuable service, and no small task, was provided by Sylvia Gaddi, supervisor of our library reference and informational services, and her staff. Sylvia bore the responsibility for researching, surveying, locating, and procuring articles and books from all over the United States, Canada, and abroad.

Dr. Martin L. Rossman, Co-Director of the Academy for Guided Imagery, and a recognized pioneer in the area of guided imagery, was kind enough to discuss and offer suggestions regarding the relaxation procedure used, and review and critique the imagery exercises in the scripts.

My appreciation goes also to my publisher, Vic Marks, and editors Sue Tauber, Rachael Preston, and Susan Juby who deserve more than a few lines of commendation for sharing my personal and professional convictions about the value of the concepts upon which this book is based, and for making this book everything it should be.

And finally, to all my patients who have suffered undue abuse, I owe a debt of gratitude for motivating me to keep on seeking, and teaching me that there is a better way for all of us to take control.

A very special thank you with love to my wife Ella for what must have seemed like endless hours laboriously spent trying to decipher and transcribe handwritten material, and for her never-ending advice, suggestions, and commentary.

REFERENCES

Ayoob, M. *The Truth About Self Protection.* New York: Bantam Books, 1983.

America Afraid: How Fear of Crime Changes the Way We Live: based on the widely publicized Figgie Report by Research & Forecasts, Inc., & Friedberg, A. New York: New American Library, 1983.

Bachman, R. "Elderly Victims." United States Department of Justice, Bureau of Justice Statistics; Washington, D.C., 1992.

Bard, M. and Sangrey, D. *The Crime Victim's Book.* New York: Basic Books, 1979.

Bart, P. *Avoiding Rape: A Study of Victims and Avoiders.* Final Report of the National Institute of Mental Health, Grant #29311, 1980.

Bart, P., and O'Brien, P.H. *Stopping Rape.* New York: Pergamon Press, 1985.

Beck, A.T. *Depression: Clinical, Experimental and Theoretical Aspects.* New York: Harper and Row, 1967.

Bennett, V., and Clagett, C. *1001 Ways to Avoid Getting Mugged, Murdered, Robbed, Raped or Ripped Off.* New York: Mason/Charter, 1977.

Benson, H. *The Relaxation Response.* New York: William Morrow and Company, Inc., 1975.

Benson, H. *Beyond the Relaxation Response.* New York: Time Books, 1984.

Biderman, A.D., et al. *Report of a Pilot Study in the District of Columbia on Victimization and Attitudes Toward Law Enforcement, Field Surveys I.* Report prepared for the President's Commission on Law Enforcement and Administration of Justice. Washington, D.C.: United States Government Printing Office, 1967.

Block, R. *Victim-Offender Dynamics in Violent Crime: Victims of Crime*—A Review of Research Issues and Method. Washington, D.C.: United States Department of Justice, 1981.

Block, R., and Skogan, W.G. *The Dynamics of Violence Between Strangers: Victim Resistance and Outcomes in Rape, Assault, and Robbery*—Final Report of the Center for Urban Affairs and Policy Research. Evanston, IL: Northwestern University, Grant #81-IJ-CX-0069, National Institute of Justice, 1984.

Brown, T., Jr., with Brown, J. *Tom Brown's Field Guide to Nature and Survival for Children.* New York: Berkley Books, 1989.

Burgess, A.W., and Holmstrom, L.L. *Rape: Victims of Crisis.* Bowie, Maryland: Robert J. Brady Co., 1974.

Castleman, M. *Crime Free.* New York: Simon and Schuster, 1984.

Check, W.A. *The Mind-Body Connection.* New York: Chelsea House Publishers, 1990.

Coates, D., Wortman, C.B., and Abbey, A. "Reactions to Victims." In Frieze, I.H., Bar-Tal, D., and Carrol, J.S. (Eds.) *New Approaches to Social Problems: Applications of Attribution Theory.* San Francisco, CA: Jossey-Bass, 1979.

Corsini, R.J. (Ed.) *Encyclopedia of Psychology.* New York: John Wiley and Sons, Vol. 2, 1984.

Cousins, N. "The Mysterious Placebo: How Mind Helps Medicine Work." *Saturday Review* (October 1, 1977): 9–16.

Davis, R. *Providing Help to Victims: A Study of Psychological and Material Outcomes.* Executive Summary—Victim Services Agency. New York: 1987.

Dejanikus, T. "New Studies Support Active Resistance to Rape." *Off Our Backs* (February 1981), Vol. II, #2, 9–23.

Dobson, T. with Shepherd-Chow, J. *Safe and Alive.* Los Angeles: J.P. Tarcher, Inc., 1984.

Dychtwald, K. *Bodymind.* New York: Pantheon Books, 1977.

Dychtwald, K. "The Powers of Mind." *New Age* (January 1978): 38–53.

Ennis, P.H. *Report of a National Survey on Criminal Victimization in the United States, Field Surveys II.* Prepared for the President's Commission on Law Enforcement and Administration and Justice. Washington, D.C.: United States Government Printing Office, 1967.

Farkas, E. and Leeds, M. *Fight Back—A Woman's Guide to Self-Defense.* New York: Holt, Rinehart and Winston, 1978.

Fattah, E.A. "Victims' Response to Confrontational Victimization: A Neglected Aspect of Victim Research." *Crime and Delinquency,* 30 #1 (January 1984), 75–89.

Federal Bureau of Investigation. *Uniform Crime Reports.* Washington, D.C.: United States Department of Justice, yearly.

Field Enterprises, Inc. Field Newspaper Syndicate, 1982.

Fighting Crime in America: An Agenda for the 1990's: A Majority Staff Report prepared for the use of the Committee on the Judiciary, United States Senate, One Hundred Second Congress, First Session, March 12, 1991.

Fike, R.A. *How to Keep From Being Robbed, Raped and Ripped Off.* Washington, D.C.: Acropolis Books, Ltd., 1983.

Frieze, I.H. "Perceptions of Battered Wives." In Frieze, I.H., Bar-Tal, D., and Carroll, J.S. (Eds.) *New Approaches to Social Problems: Applications of Attribution Theory.* San Francisco, CA: Jossey-Bass, 1979.

Gardner, Carol B. "Safe Conduct: Women, Crime and Self in Public Places." *Social Problems,* Vol. 37, #3, 311–328 (August 1990).

Garofalo, J. "The Fear of Crime: Causes and Consequences." In *Victims of Crime. A Review of Research Issues and Methods.* Washington, D.C.: United States Department of Justice, 1981.

Gilbert, N. "The Phantom Epidemic of Sexual Assault." *The Public Interest.* Washington, D.C.: National Affairs, Inc., #103 (Spring 1991)

Gilmartin, B.G. "The Case Against Spanking." *Human Behavior,* Vol. 8, #2, 18–23 (February 1979).

Gottfredson, M.R. "On the Etiology of Criminal Victimization." In *Victims of Crime—Review of Research Issues and Methods.* Washington, D.C.: United States Department of Justice, 1981.

Grayson, B., and Stein, M.I. "Attracting Assault: Victims' Nonverbal Cues." *Journal of Communication,* 68–75 (Winter 1981).

Harlow, C.W. *Female Victims of Violent Crime.* Washington, D.C.: United States Department of Justice (January 1991).

Hazelwood, R.R., and Burgess, A.W. (Eds.) *Practical Aspects of Rape Investigation.* New York: Elsevier Science Publishing Co., Inc., 1987.

Hazelwood, R.R., Reboussin, R. and Warren, J.I. "Serial Rape: Correlates of Increased Aggression and the Relationship of Offender Pleasure to Victim Resistance." *Journal of Interpersonal Violence,* Vol. 4, #1, 65–78 (March 1989).

Hindelang, M.J., Gottfredson, M.R., and Garofalo, J. *Victims of Personal Crime: An Empirical Foundation for a Theory of Personal Victimization.* Cambridge, MA: Ballinger Publishing Co., 1978.

Hinsie, L.E., and Campbell, R.J. *Psychiatric Dictionary.* New York: Oxford University Press, 1960.

Holub, K. "A Case of Rape." *West Magazine, San Jose Mercury News* (October 21, 1990): 16–27.

Hugick, L. "Public Sees Crime Up Nationally." *Gallup Poll News Service,* Vol. 56, #43a (March 1992).

Human Behavior. Vol. 7, #12, 60 (November 1978).

Hursch, C.J. *The Trouble With Rape.* Chicago: Nelson-Hall, 1977.

Innes, C.A., and Greenfield, L.A. *Violent State Prisoners and Their Victims.* Washington, D.C.: United States Department of Justice, Office of Justice Programs, Bureau of Justice Statistics, Special Report (July 1990).

Jacobson, E. *Progressive Relaxation.* Chicago: University of Chicago Press, 1974.

Janoff-Bulman, R. "Esteem and Control Bases of Blame: 'Adaptive' Strategies for Victims Versus Observers." *Journal of Personality,* 50, 180–192 (1982).

Janoff-Bulman, R., and Lang-Gunn, L. "Coping With Disease and Accidents: The Role of Self-Blame Attributions." In Abramson, L.Y. (Ed.) *Social-Personal Inference in Clinical Psychology.* New York: the Guilford Press, 1983.

Kabat-Zinn, J. *Full Catastrophe Living.* New York: Delacorte Press, Bantam Doubleday Dell Publishing Group, 1990.

Kagan, J., and Havemann, E. *Psychology: An Introduction.* New York: Harcourt Brace Jovanovich, 1972.

Kahn, A.S. (Ed.) *Final Report. American Psychological Association Task Force on the Victims of Crime and Violence,* 1984.

Keene, K.H., and Ladd, E.C. (Eds.) "Public Opinion and Demographic Report." In *The American Enterprise.* Washington, D.C.: The American Enterprise Institute for Public Policy Research, Vol. 2, #4 (July/August, 1991).

Kidd, B., and McCluggage, D. "Secrets of Visualization." *Skiing* (March 1991): 20–21.

Kidder, L.H., Boell, J.L., and Moyer, M.M. "Rights Consciousness and Victimization Prevention: Personal Defense and Assertiveness Training." *Journal of Social Issues,* Vol. 39 (2), 153–168 (1983).

Klaus, P.A., Kaplan, C.G., Rand, M.R., and Taylor, B.M. "The Victim." In *Report to the Nation on Crime and Justice,* Zawitz, M.W. (Ed.). Washington, D.C.: United States Department of Justice, 1988.

Klaus, P.A., Kaplan, C.G., Rand, M.R., Taylor, B.M., Zawitz, M.W., and Smith, S.E. "The Criminal Event." In *Report to the Nation on Crime and Justice,* Zawitz, M.W. (Ed.). Washington, D.C.: United States Department of Justice, 1983.

Krech, D., and Crutchfield, R.S. *Elements of Psychology.* New York: Alfred A. Knopf, 1958.

Landsberg, M. "As Crime Fear Rises, More Women Learning to Handle Firearms." *The Record,* February 8, 1993.

McIntyre, J.J. *Rape, Resistance and Injury: A Follow-Up Study.* Final Report of the National Institute of Mental health, Grant #39176. Washington, D.C.: National Institute of Mental Health (1987).

McIntyre, J.J. *Victim Response to Rape: Alternative Outcomes.* Final Report of Mental Health Grant #29045, National Institute of Mental Health, 1980.

McIntyre, J.J, Myint, T., and Curtis, L. *Sexual Assault Outcomes—Abstract,* Grant #29045-02. Washington, D.C.: The National Institute of Mental Health (1977–89).

McManus, J., Editor-in-Chief. *Powers of Healing.* Alexandria, VA: Time-Life Books, 1989.

Malamuth, N.M. "Rape Proclivity Among Males." *The Journal of Social Issues,* 37 (4), 138–157 (1981).

Mattera, J. *The Power of Your Subconscious Mind.* Englewood Cliffs, N.J.: Prentice-Hall, Inc., 1963.

Meier, B. "Reality and Anxiety: Crime and Fear of It." *The New York Times,* February 18, 1993.

Murphy, M. *The Future of the Body.* Los Angeles, CA: J.P. Tarcher, Inc., 1992.

Murphy, M., and White, R.A. *The Psychic Side of Sports.* Reading, MA: Addison-Wesley Publishing Co., 1978.

National Update. Washington, D.C.: United States Department of Justice, Bureau of Justice Statistics; July, 1992; Vol. II, (1).

National Victim Center. "Male Rape." *Infolink.* Fort Worth, Texas: Vol. 1, #37, 1992.

Newcomb, T.M. *Social Psychology.* New York: The Dryden Press, 1950.

Ornish, D. *Dr. Dean Ornish's Program for Reversing Heart Disease.* New York: Random House, 1990.

Pava, W.S. Bateman, P., Appleton, M.K., and Glascock, J. "Self-Defense Training for Visually Impaired Women." *Journal of Visual Impairment and Blindness* (December 1991).

Perloff, L.S. "Perceptions of Vulnerability to Victimization." *Journal of Social Issues,* 39 (2), 41–61 (1983).

Porter, K., and Foster, J. *Visual Athletics.* Dubuque, IA: William C. Brown Publishers, 1990.

Queen's Bench Foundation. *Rape Prevention and Resistance.* San Francisco, CA: 1976.

Quinsey, V.L., and Upfold, D. "Rape Completion and Victim Injury as a Function of Female Resistance Strategy." *Canadian Journal of Behavioural Science/Revue.* Canadienne Des Sciences Du Comportement, 17 (1), 40–50 (1985).

Rape in America: A Report to the Nation. Virginia: National Victim Center, 1992.

Reiss, A. *Studies in Crime and Law Enforcement in Major Metropolitan Areas.* President's Commission on Law Enforcement and Administration of Justice, Field Surveys III. Washington, D.C.: United States Government Printing Office, 1967.

Richards, L. "A Theoretical Analysis of Nonverbal Communication and Victim Selection for Sexual Assault." *Clothing and Textiles Research Journal.* Summer, 1991; Vol. 9, (4), 55–64.

Ross, H.W. and Richman, L. "The Criminal Victimization of the Physically Challenged." Draft, Grant-in-Aid, San Diego State University, 1986.

Rossman, M.L. *Healing Yourself.* New York: Pocket Books, a Division of Simon and Schuster, Inc., 1987.

Samuels, M., and Samuels, N. *Seeing With the Mind's Eye.* New York: Random House, Inc., 1975.

Sanders, W.B. *Rape and Women's Identity.* Beverly Hills, CA: Sage Publications, 1980.

Scherer, Migael. *Still Loved by the Sun.* New York: Simon and Schuster, 1992.-

Schneider, A.L. "Methodological Problems in Victim Surveys and Their Implications for Research in Victimology. In *Victims of Crime—A Review of Research Issues and Method.* Washington, D.C.: United States Department of Justice, 1981.

Shone, R. *Creative Visualization.* Rochester, VT: Destiny Books, 1988.

Siegel, B. *Love, Medicine and Miracles.* New York: Harper and Row, 1986.

Skogan, W.G., and Maxfield, M.G. *Coping With Crime.* Beverly Hills, CA: Sage Publications, Inc., Vol. 124, 1981.

Sparks, R.F. "Multiple Victimization: Evidence, Theory and Future Research." In *Victims of Crime, A Review of Research Issues and Method.* Washington, D.C.: United States Department of Justice, 1981.

Sparks, R.F., Genn, H., and Dodd, D. *Surveying Victims.* New York: John Wiley, 1977.

"Statistical Analysis Center Edition of the Illinois Crime Report Data. Table: Rape and Attempted Rape Offenses in Chicago Standard Metropolitan Statistical Area, 1972–1980." In Bart, P.B. and O'Brien, P.H., *Stopping Rape.* New York: Pergamon Press, Inc., 1985.

Stedman, T.L. *Stedman's Medical Dictionary, 24th Edition.* Baltimore, MD: Williams and Wilkins, 1982.

Storaska, F. *How to Say No to a Rapist and Survive.* New York: Random House, 1975.

Symonds, P.M. *Dynamic Psychology.* New York: Appelton—Century—Crofts, Inc., 1949.

Teich, M. "Picture This." *American Health* (June 1990): 71.

Toby, J. "Violence in School." In Tonry, M.H., and Morris, N. (Eds.) *Crime and Justice.* The University of Chicago Press (1983), Vol. 4.

Tyiska, C.G. "Responding to Disabled Victims of rime." *NOVA Newsletter*, 8–12. Washington, D.C., 1990.

Victims of Crime—An Overview. Washington, D.C.: United States Department of Justice, November, 1987.

Violent Death in America: 1991's Record Murder Toll: A Majority Staff Report Prepared for the use of the Committee on the Judiciary, United States Senate, One Hundred Second Congress, Second Session, January, 1992.

Warshaw, R. *I Never Called It Rape.* New York: Harper and Row, 1988.

Weil, A. *Natural Health, Natural Medicine.* Boston: Houghton Mifflin Company, 1990.

Weinstein, N.D. "Unrealistic Optimism About Future Life Events." *Journal of Personality and Social Psychology*, 39, 806–820 (1980).

Whittmore, G. *Street Wisdom for Women.* Boston: Quinlan Press, 1986.

Wilson, K., Faison, R., and Britton, G.M. "Cultural Aspects of Male Sex Aggression." *Deviant Behavior*, 4, 241–255 (1983).

Wortman, C.B., and Dintzer, L., "Is An Attributional Analysis of the Learned Helplessness Phenomenon Viable? A Critique of the Abramson-Seligman-Teasdale Reformulation." *Journal of Abnormal Psychology*, 87, 75–90 (1978).

Wright, R. "Rape and Physical Violence." In West, D.J. (Ed.) *Sex Offenders in the Criminal Justice System.* Cambridge, England: Cropwood Conference Series, 1980.

Zawitz, M.W., Gaskins, C.K., Koppel, H., Greenfield, L.A., and Greenwood, P. "The Response to Crime." In *Report to the Nation on Crime and Justice*, Zawitz, M.W. (Ed.). Washington, D.C.: United States Department of Justice, 1988.

Zoucha-Jenson, J.M. and Coyne, A. "The Effects of Resistance Strategies on Rape." *American Journal of Public Health*, Vol. 83, #11 (November 1993).

Index